Advance praise for *The Healing Powers of Olive Oil*

"Olive oil is one of our important foods. This book deserves to be in everybody's home library."
　　—Elson Haas, M.D., author of *Staying Healthy with Nutrition, 21st Century Edition*

"A fascinating read about olive oil's secret ingredients."
　　—Chef Ann Cooper, author of *Lunch Lessons: Changing the Way We Feed Our Children*

"This is a landmark book full of entertaining anecdotes which explains the olive oil and health connection."
　　—Jan McBarron, M.D., cohost of *Duke and the Doctor Radio Show*

"Orey's book brings the best and highly practical information about the core of the longevity-boosting Mediterranean diet—olive oil."
　　—Karlis Ullis, M.D., Medical Director of Sports Medicine and Anti-Aging Medical Group of Santa Monica, California

THE HEALING POWERS OF
Olive Oil

A Complete Guide to Nature's Liquid Gold

CAL OREY

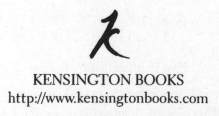

KENSINGTON BOOKS
http://www.kensingtonbooks.com

KENSINGTON BOOKS are published by
Kensington Publishing Corp.
850 Third Avenue
New York, NY 10022

ISBN-13: 978-0-7582-2221-3
ISBN-10: 0-7582-2221-1

First Printing: February 2008
10 9 8 7 6 5 4 3 2 1

Printed in the United States of America

CONTENTS

Foreword

I spend my time traveling in the exciting world of olive oil, tasting and enjoying olive oil as I go. From Tuscany to Sicily and Catalonia to Andalusia, the unique tastes and flavours of the extra virgin olive oils never cease to amaze me.

This year, the pungently herbaceous oils of Croatia are competing in my kitchen with the tropical fruit tones of oils from Cordoba and Seville. And as the year unfolds, I will be adding Southern Hemisphere olive oils from Chile and Australia.

In the Mediterranean region, this wonderful product has always been an integral part of the culture. It is used extensively in the kitchen and at the table. Its consumption starts at breakfast with a slice of toast rubbed with fresh-cut tomato and drizzled with olive oil, and continues through all the meals of the day.

Everyone here knows that extra virgin olive oil is not just a cooking medium but a flavouring ingredient in its own right. They also know of its health benefits and healing properties. Whether it is a case of sunburn, persistent earache, or dry hair, they have traditionally turned to olive oil.

Now, new research highlighting the beneficial qualities of extra virgin olive oil not only confirms these uses but adds a whole host of other beneficial effects from its use. Whether it is coronary heart disease, diabetes, bad digestion, or age-related deterioration, olive oil has been shown to be beneficial in its prevention and treatment.

In this new book, *The Healing Powers of Olive Oil*, Cal Orey brings together ancient folklore and modern research to show you how to get the best from olive oil.

—Judy Ridgway, author of
*Judy Ridgway's Best Olive Oil Buys
Round the World,*
www.oliveoil.uk.com

Acknowledgments

I admit it. I don't like to cook, nor have I been to Europe—my unful-
filled dream since I was a kid. Thanks to this book, I got my trip to
Spain, Italy, and Greece—vicariously through the chefs, olive oil producers, and other olive oil experts who live in the Mediterranean basin
or who have traveled to European countries. But I am truly happy to
be a Northern California native, and I live about 150 miles away from
where enthusiastic olive oil growers are plentiful and their extraordinary olive oil is in demand.

While I have been tagged a health author, I confess I wasn't always
an olive oil lover. I didn't know porcini olive oil from citrus olive oil,
nor that Spain is the largest olive oil producer in the world. But I was
an eager student. And, I want to give credit to the savvy medical doctors, nutritionists, and Italian pioneers of olive oil who shared their
worldy knowledge. I won't forget the busy California olive oil producers during harvest time in the fall when they took time out to help me
with this challenging and enlightening project.

I must give credit to my two down-to-earth Northern California
friends—Kim Barrow and geologist Jim Berkland—who appreciate the

ground of our Golden State, and who gave me grounded support as I entered olive land.

This morning, I sit in my study in the soft light of an olive oil lamp, drinking chamomile tea from an olive-painted ceramic mug. I just took a shower with heavenly lavender-scented olive oil-based soap, applied a dab of extra virgin olive oil on my two Brittanys' coats (Simon, 3 1/2 years old, and Seth, 5 months old, were on their best behavior during my research and writing of this book), and spritzed my happy houseplants with olive oil and water. Earlier, I fixed scrambled eggs, spraying the frying pan with olive oil, with thanks to a gifted Italian cook—Gemma Sciabica. And, I am thankful that I have learned from this olive oil guru of the twentieth century that I *can* bake with olive oil.

As the months passed during my research for *The Healing Powers of Olive Oil*, I began to change like a caterpillar turning into a butterfly. Blame my transformation on all the interesting people I crossed paths with, from an olive oil farmer in Umbria to Frantoio's chef Duilio Valenti from Milan, who made me a vegetarian brick-oven pizza with basil, tomatoes, and olive oil.

I thank my editor, Richard Ember, who planted the idea of this book in my brain and allowed me to write it. And, like a sporting dog, I retrieved the new project with passion, energy, and a genuine desire to learn about the wide, wide world of olive oil, once called liquid gold by Homer.

In an olive seed pit, I got to telecommute around the globe. The best part is, as a health-conscious baby boomer (a person born between 1946 and 1964), I now have a new relationship with olive oil and its powerful virtues. Chances are I will be both happier and healthier in the years to come. Plus, when I do go to Europe (and I will), I will appreciate its precious olive oil and hardworking producers. Lastly, I know now in my heart that this book was meant to be written by me—for you. A toast to olive oil, the twenty-first century elixir that is as good as it gets.

PART 1

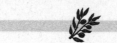

A TIME FOR OLIVE OIL

The Power of Olive Oil

Except the vine, there is no plant which bears a
fruit as of great importance as the olive.
—Pliny[1]

In the fifties, I grew up in San Jose, California, a place once known for its plentiful prune tree orchards. Today, as a nature-loving Northern Californian who currently lives amid tall pine trees in South Lake Tahoe, I was pleasantly surprised to discover that within three hours of my mountain-style home—with rolling hills much like in Italy, Spain, and Greece—olive groves are growing and people are producing olive oil, known as liquid gold, in a Mediterranean-type weather in the Golden State.

When I was in my late twenties, it was my dream to go to Europe. I dog-eared one of those Europe-on-a-shoestring-budget travel books and planned my trip. But I opted to go to graduate school instead. So, I never got to enjoy the exotic Mediterranean countries or taste the European cuisine—including its wide world of olive oil.

The closest I've come to Italy, the second largest producer of olive oil, is by watching the film *Under the Tuscan Sun*, which is about a divorced writing professor and book reviewer—played by Diane Lane— and based loosely on a novel created by Frances Mayes, who taught classes at my alumni college, San Francisco State University. With envy, I viewed her protagonist, Frances, learning to live and laugh again thousands of miles away from the San Francisco Bay Area. In Tuscany, where she relocates, it's the eccentric, down-to-earth locals and observing an earthy harvest of olives (right outside her new home) that finds a place in her heart.

In the real world, I sit here in my study with snow-covered ground outdoors in the California Sierras and fantasize about how wonderful it would be to live in Italy amid olive trees. But, whisking off in a plane to Europe isn't going to happen for me today or tomorrow. Still, I will take you along with me to visit real people and real places where you will get a real flavor of the Mediterranean basin and of the healing powers of olive oil.

THE OLIVE YIELDS A POWERFUL OIL

Olive oil has been praised by people as one of Mother Nature's most healthful fats, especially if it is extra virgin olive oil. And now, olive oil—and other healing oils—are making the news worldwide, and are here to stay in homes, restaurants, and even fast-food chains.

People from all walks of life—including some olive oil pioneers and contemporary medical experts—believe olive oil helps fight body fat and keeps blood pressure down as well as heart disease at bay. Olive oil is also known to help relieve colds and maintain healthy skin.

Jean Carper, a leading authority on health and nutrition, points out that new Italian research finds olive oil contains antioxidants, similar to those in tea and red wine, that fight heart disease, including LDL cholesterol's ability to clog arteries.[2]

Dietician and nutrition consultant Pat Baird, author of *The Pyramid Cookbook: Pleasures of the Food Guide Pyramid*, touts the golden liquid, too. "I love the whole idea of olive oil's versatility. I use it for baking, as well as salad dressings and sautéing. Olive oil has been around for a long time, and the more we know about it, the more we learn about its great contribution to good health."[3]

Liz Applegate, Ph.D., a renowned health, nutrition, and fitness expert, wrote in her book *101 Miracle Foods That Heal Your Heart*, "Rich in history, and even richer in heart-healthy benefits, olive oil is the 'king' of oils."[4]

Health-Boosting Nutrients in Extra Virgin Olive Oil

Medical researchers around the world continue to find new health-promoting nutrients in olives and olive oil. Here are some of the nutrients in extra virgin olive oil:

Vitamin E: an antioxidant vitamin that can help strengthen immune responses and reduces the risk of heart disease and some forms of cancer.

Essential Fatty Acids: good-for-you fats such as the omega-3s and omega-6s that can help stave off heart disease, obesity, and diabetes.

Chlorophyll: a substance that has antioxidant properties.

Phenol Compounds: substances that also act as antioxidants.

Phytoestrogens: substances that may help beat bone loss and minimize pesky symptoms of menopause.

Sterols: substances that counter the intestinal absorption of cholesterol in foods.

Most important, like apple cider and red wine vinegars, extra virgin olive oil contains polyphenols, naturally occurring compounds that act as powerful antioxidants (disease-fighting enzymes that protect your body by trapping free-radical molecules and getting rid of them before damage occurs).

OLIVE OILS WITH POLYPHENOLS

Keep in mind, if you're a health-conscious person like I am, you'll quickly ask, "Which olive oil has the highest polyphenols?"

"Phenol content is determined by olive variety, time of picking, olive condition and processing method, whether the oil is refined, and the length of time the oil has been treated," explains Dr. John Deane, an internal medicine specialist in Marin County, California, and an olive oil expert who writes for *The Olive Oil Source* newsletter.

That said, it's the Tuscan varieties, points out Deane, such as Coratina, Frantoio, Lucca, and Pendolino, that boast the highest good-for-you poly-phenols. "These oils are valuable in that when blended with a low poly-phenol oil, they will extend the shelf life by preventing rancidity," he adds.

The olive oil master also says that the bulk of olive oil we consume in America comes from Italy and Spain. But the glitch is, that means it's most likely refined—and lower in phenols.

So, what do you do if you're on a mission to get an olive oil that is polyphenol-rich? According to Deane, if you choose a brand that reads "extra virgin," boasts the California Olive Oil Council (COOC) seal, is from the "current harvest season," and has been properly stored, you should be holding a healthful bottle of olive oil, like a good bottle of antioxidant-rich wine, with polyphenols.

Another interesting note I discovered is that olive oils that are higher in polyphenols tend to be harsher, bitter, and stronger flavored. That makes me think of dark chocolate. It is not as sweet and mellow as milk chocolate. But then, it's the darker chocolate that contains the heart-healthy antioxidants, right? And, like other healthful foods, such as olive oil, sometimes it takes a while to acquire a taste for them.

OLIVE OIL BASICS 101

Olive oil, one of the oldest vegetable oils, comes from the fruit of the olive tree (*Olea europae L.*), which was originally found in the Mediterranean basin. It has been used since biblical times in cooking, as a medicinal agent, in cosmetics, in soaps, and even as fuel for lamps.

So, what exactly is olive oil, anyhow?

> **Olive Oil:** oil pressed from olives, used in salad dressings, for cooking, as an ingredient in soaps, and as an emollient.
> —*The American Heritage Dictionary*

Olive oil can be made from a wide variety of olives, such as black and green olives, and other types. "There are at least 30 olive varieties used extensively for olive oil and then add another 100 or so depending on where you are. In total 300 plus varieties," explains Judy Ridgway. Of course, I have learned that this number varies depending on your olive oil reference source.

The following kinds of olives—including the polyphenol-rich ones—used for olive oils are listed from A to Z.

OLIVE POTPOURRI

Kind	Olives Grown From	Olive Oil Taste
Arbequina	Puglia, Italy	Fresh and fruity
Barnea	Australia, Israel, New Zealand	Sweet almonds, sometimes with a banana flavor
Biancollia	Sicily	Herbal tomatoes
Cerasuolo	Sicily	Apples, sweet herbs, and tomatoes
Cornatina	Carato (near Barl) and Puglia, Italy	Fruity, bitter, and peppery with a tinge of sweet taste; high in polyphenols
Cornicabra	Spain	Light bitterness, peppery, and fruit notes; younger oils pungent, smooth, like an almond aftertaste
Frantoio	Tuscany, Italy; Argentina; Chile; California; New Zealand; Australia	Fruity, aromatic, and a peppery taste; late bloomers soft, almost sweet, like a mild almond flavor
Galega	Portugal	Fruity smell, soft, smooth flavor of green fruit and grass with a taste of almonds

Kind	Olives Grown From	Olive Oil Taste
Hojblanca	Andalusia, Spain	Often sweet, and a bit fruity, followed by a mild peppery taste; a lingering bitter aftertaste of fruit
Kalamata	Kalamata, Greece	Distinct taste
Koroneiki	Koroni, Greece	Fruity, touch of green apple, fresh, grassy flavor
La Tanche	Nyons, Provence, France; Sicily	Sweet apples and herbs
Leccino	Tuscany, Umbria, Lazio, Italy	Bland, a bit fruity, not bitter or peppery, a little sweetness
Maurino	Central Italy and California	Bitter herbs with nuts and pepper
Mission	California	Fruity, more peppery and bitter than Cornicabra oils, thick, a hint of almond sweetness
Moraiolo	Central Italy	Herbaceous with bitter nuts and pepper
Nocellara Del Belice	Castelvetrano, Italy	Fresh and delightful flavor
Ogilarolo	Puglia, Italy	Sweet nuts and light apples
Olivastra	Tuscany and Slovenia	Creamy apples and herbs
Peranzana	Southern Italy	Herbs and bitter salad leaves

Kind	Olives Grown From	Olive Oil Taste
Picholine	France	Lacks bitterness, mild, almost sweet
Picual	Spain	Distinct [butter] and strong taste like "figs and wet wood"; high polyphenols
Picudo	Spain	Smooth, strong, and distinctive taste; sweet; grassy first; strong aroma of bitter citrus; low levels of polyphenols
Taggiasca	Liguria, Italy	Sweet apples, nuts, and light herbs
Tonda Iblea	Sicily	Crushed tomatoes

Sources: Judy Ridgway and *The Olive Oil Companion*.

THE ART OF PRODUCTION

From harvesting to bottling, the time and tender loving care put into nature's olives and making premium quality olive oil is the same today as it was centuries ago. The bulk of olive oil is made in Mediterranean countries such as Spain, Italy, and Greece, with a small percentage produced in California, Australia, parts of South America, and other countries.

Harvesting: Varying from region to region, olive harvests usually take place between mid-November and mid-January. During this time, olive oil producers are much like writers on deadline—busy, excited, and did I say busy? The olives are collected in nets that are placed around the foot of the tree (see the film *Under the Tuscan Sun* to get a visual image), and within 24 hours of harvest, the olives are taken directly to a mill to be pressed into olive oil.

Pressing: An olive paste is created by crushing the whole fruit (yes, including the pits that you spit out when munching on your favorite olives). This is usually done under granite or steel millstones that resemble those used more than 1,000 years ago. The paste is then spread onto thin mats, which are stacked and placed into a machine press. As the press applies several hundred pounds of pressure, oil and water seep out of the mats and drip into collection vats. This process requires no heat—hence the term "first cold-pressed" olive oil.

A bit confused about the term "cold press," let alone "first," I contacted food-science columnist Robert L. Wolke, professor emeritus of chemistry at the University of Pittsburgh and author of *What Einstein Told His Cook: Kitchen Science Explained* (W.W. Norton & Company, 2005). He gave me the lowdown on cold-pressing semantics: "Cold pressed means that the olives or the press are not heated or treated with hot water. The maximum allowed temperature for extra virgin oil is 25°C or 77°F. Heat would give a higher yield of oil during the pressing, but would compromise the quality and flavor. But that 'cold' or unheated pressing is the only pressing. The olives are virtually never pressed a second time at higher pressure, which would just squeeze bitter juices out of the pits. Instead, the remaining oil is coaxed out with hot water or an organic solvent. That oil, however, is a lower quality and cannot be labeled 'extra virgin.' Still, producers like to claim 'first pressing' for their extra virgin oils. It just sounds impressive."

Other methods, I learned, are also sometimes used to extract oil from olives. One is centrifugation. "A centrifuge spins materials around rapidly, like the spin cycle on a washing machine," explains Wolke. "After the pressing, it separates oil from the watery juices." However, mechanical pressing is the most popular way.

After pressing, the oil is then left to settle, and any vegetable water is removed by centrifuge machines. When the olive oil is created, it is set aside to be evaluated for its quality and categorized.

GRADES OF OLIVE OIL

Extra virgin: Extracted from the highest-quality olives. It must have less than 1 percent natural acidity. Its "fruity" flavor is intense and great in salads.

Virgin: Processed mechanically (using pressure) and without heat, which changes the oil's acidity to 1 to 5 percent. It's recommended for use in salad dressings and marinades.

Pure: A mix of refined olive oil (treated with steam and chemicals) and virgin oils. Its acidity ranges from 3 to 4 percent. Less costly, it's most often used in cooking.

Extracted and refined: Made from whole cull olives and extracted during a second pressing with a chemical solvent; virgin oil is added for flavor.

Pomace: Made by a chemical extraction of the residue left over after the crushing and second pressing of the olives. It contains 5 to 10 percent acidity; virgin oil is added for flavor.

All-Natural Processing

Olive oil expert Dr. Deane confirms that extra virgin olive is one of the few oils that can be consumed and enjoyed without chemical processing. "Fresh pressed olive oil can be eaten immediately, and retains the natural flavors, vitamins, minerals, antioxidants, and other healthy products of the ripe olive fruit," he notes.

THE DA VINCI DECODED LABELS LEXICON

Terms to Know	Definition	The Real Deal
Blended olive oil	Combination of various olive types, regions, and countries	Grocery store brands are often blended
Imported from Italy	Gives the impression that the olives were grown in Italy	The fact is, the oil was bottled there
100 percent pure olive oil	A quality found in retail grocery stores	Better grades include "virgin" on the label
Made from refined olive oils	Hints that the essence is inside the bottle	In reality, the taste and acidity were chemically produced
Light olive oil	Insinuates a low fat content	The term points to a lighter color, not

Terms to Know	Definition	The Real Deal
		fewer calories or less fat
From hand-picked olives	Suggests that Mom and Pop gave the olives personal TLC	Vague about the harvest method—hands-on or tree-shaking
First cold press	Implies this is the number-one oil that came from the first press of the olives	The key word is "cold," because if heat is used, the olive oil's chemistry is changed

Sources: Wikipedia, The Olive Oil Source.

THE OLIVE CITY

Before I spread my wings and take you to meet olive experts worldwide and discover olive oils, I want to reiterate that I never knew that olives have been growing in California for centuries. Nor did I know that California's Corning, coined the Olive City, is home to the Bell Carter Olive Company, the world's largest ripe olive cannery. But while there are at least 300 varieties of olives grown from Oroville to Modesto in California, the Mission and Manzanillo are the most commonly used for olive oil.

FUN FACTS ABOUT CALIFORNIA RIPE OLIVES

You see them all the time. They're in many of your favorite foods and recipes—or maybe you like to eat them all by themselves. But how much do you know about California Ripe Olives?

Olives are a member of the fruit family.	Olives grow on trees and may have been first cultivated over 5,000 years ago in Syria and Crete.

In the 1700s, monks brought olives to Mexico and then to California by way of missions. The first cuttings were planted in 1769 at the San Diego Mission.

Today, anywhere from 80,000 to 106,000 tons of olives are produced in California each year.

About 70 to 80 percent of all ripe olives are grown in California's approximately 35,000 acres.

Olive trees bloom each year in May, and by mid-September, the olives are ready to be picked.

Olives, as they come from the tree, are too bitter to eat, so they are cured.

Four main varieties of olives are grown in California:

Mission—originally cultivated by the Franciscan missions.

Manzanillo—the most prevalent.

Sevillano—the larger size.

Ascolano—the larger size.

Commercial cultivation of California olives began in the late 1800s.

California Ripe Olives grow in a variety of sizes: small, medium, large, extra large, jumbo, colossal, and super colossal.

Olive trees tend to alternate their yields, producing large crops one year and smaller crops the next.

Olives destined for canneries are picked when they are still green and then become Ripe Olives.

Black ripe olives are oxidized, during processing; they are never dyed.

Source: California Olive Industry, www.calolive.org.

Medical doctors, nutritionists, olive oil producers and manufacturers, chefs, and consumers are now learning what people during biblical times practiced. True, in past centuries it was not known exactly how or why olive oil had healing powers—but it did. It's clear as a bottle of freshly harvested olive oil that peasants to royalty knew that olive oil had versatile virtues, worked wonders, and was as good as gold.

THE GOLDEN SECRETS TO REMEMBER

New research shows that olive oil, especially polyphenol-rich extra virgin olive oil, which is made from a variety of olives in the Mediterranean countries—as well as from other places around the globe—may help you to:

✓ Lower your risk of heart disease and cancer.
✓ Enhance your immune system.
✓ Prevent cancer.
✓ Stave off diabetes.
✓ Fight fat.
✓ Slow the aging process.
✓ Add years to your life.

Most important, the quality of olive oil matters for your health's sake. Natural, organic, and cold pressed are recommended by olive oil producers to medical doctors.

In this book, I will show you how using olive oil (and other healing oils) is one of the best things you can do for yourself—and your health. But note, many people will not want to reap the benefits of olive oil by swallowing a tablespoon (or two) solo. While olive oil is great on salads, it also is a great seasoning for many foods. Olive oil has a vast number of uses in cooking, and I've included more than 50 recipes to help heal your body, mind, and spirit. And the versatile oil can do so much more.

But first, let's go way, way back into the past. Take a close-up look at why and how olive oil is one of the world's first—and most prized—natural medicines.

A Genesis of the Olive

The olive tree is surely the richest gift of Heaven, I can scarcely expect bread.
—Thomas Jefferson[1]

The art of using olive oil for physical and mental well-being goes back 6,000 years. As early as 400 B.C., Hippocrates, "the father of medicine," used olive oil in over 60 therapeutic remedies to treat his patients. In the era of the Romans and Egyptians, olive oil was mixed with herbs for medicinal treatments. Olive oil has been more than just a food to the people of the Mediterranean—it has been a medicinal agent and antibiotic, and has even provided promises of vitality, strength, and much more. Century after century, people discovered that the golden liquid works wonders for health.[2]

Today, nutritionists and researchers around the world continue to find more and more powerful uses for this universal oil. And history shows that people since biblical times have taken advantage not only of the internal benefits of olive oil, but of its external perks as well.

Olive oil's great power is timeless. The earliest historical record of olive oil appears to be when Homer, the legendary early Greek poet, called olive oil "liquid gold" in the famous work the *Odyssey*. In ancient Greece, athletes rubbed it from head to toe. Not only did the golden liquid illuminate alive and beautiful bodies, but it was also used on the dead bodies of saints and heroes in their tombs.

HEALING OILS IN BIBLICAL TIMES

The olive tree was praised as the most valuable and versatile tree during the biblical era. Oil is mentioned 191 times in the Bible; seven of these times refer to olive oil, but in 147 of the references to oil, olive oil can be inferred by the reader, according to the *Healing Oils of the Bible*'s author, David Stewart, Ph.D.[3]

He explains, "When olive oil was extracted in Biblical times, the whole fruit was crushed by a stone wheel (as at Gethsemane) or mashed by treading under foot (as in Micah 6:5). The broken olives were placed in special baskets where the oil was allowed to drain into vats or basins by the force of gravity. This could take a few hours or a day or two. In the Bible, the resulting product was called 'first oil,' 'beaten oil,' or 'fine oil.' (Numbers 28:5)"[4]

Adds Stewart, "In today's language we call this 'virgin oil.' The oil that drains in the first hour or so is called 'extra virgin,' while that which drains later is simply called 'virgin.'"[5]

One of the most unforgettable references to olive oil and its remarkable healing powers is in the parable of the Good Samaritan who tends to a beaten and robbed traveler. The cure-all for treating the down-and-out individual's wounds is simply with oil and wine.

Here are some other interesting biblical references to the olive leaf, fruit, and tree. These were gleaned from a variety of sources all leading to the Bible:

- "His branches shall spread, and his beauty shall be as the olive tree." (Hosea 14:6)
- "Mount of Olives—so called because of the olive trees that cover its sides, is a mountain ridge to the east of Jerusalem. (1 Kings 11:7; Ezek. 11:23; Zech. 14:4)
- For the Lord thy God bringeth thee into a good land, a land of brooks of water, of fountains and depths that spring out of valleys and hills; a land of wheat, and barley, and vines, and fig trees, and pomegranates; a land of olive trees and honey." (Deuteronomy 8:7–9)

In many regions, it's believed that the news of the end of the great flood was delivered by a single dove carrying one green olive tree branch in its beak. Later, the vivid image of that dove with the olive branch became the symbol of peace around the world. A reference in the Bible states: "And the dove came in to him in the evening, and lo, in her mouth was an olive leaf plucked off. So Noah knew that the waters were abated from off the earth." (Genesis 8:11)

Not only has it been noted that Christian missionaries brought the olive tree with them for food as well as religious ceremonies, but olive oil was also believed to be the oil of choice to anoint the kings of the Greeks and the Jews.

While the people in biblical times may have been clueless as to why olive oil had healing powers, they considered it a valuable staple in meals and used it both in cooking and on the table.

Since that period, olive oil is no longer the stuff of folk medicine and old wives' tales. Modern science is proving that folk healers were right all along. Both then and now, the precious oil is touted for its versatile uses and healthful properties, for the total body, mind, and spirit.

And, of course, the olive tree—the source of the sacred olive—is not to be ignored. Roman mythology attributes the birth of healing olives to Hercules, who struck the ground and caused an olive tree to sprout.[6] But there's more . . .

ODE TO THE OLIVE TREE

The olive tree has a long, long history of proving its value to people around the world since biblical times. It is mentioned in both the Old Testament and Greek mythology. It's been noted as the symbol of wisdom and peace.

Remember Athena, the legendary goddess of Greece? While Roman mythology links the olive tree to Hercules, the sacred olive is also connected to the goddess Athena and Athens. As the legend goes, Zeus had decreed that the city should be given to the god who offered the most useful gift to the people. Poseidon gave them the horse. Athena struck the bare soil with her spear and caused an olive tree to spring up. The people were so happy with the olive that Zeus gave the city to Athena and named it Athens after her.[7]

In the past, olive trees were recognized as sturdy and priceless. Olive tree leaves, fruit, and oil have been touted for centuries for their variety of health virtues, from healing properties to antiaging benefits.

So where exactly does the variety of tree (*Olea europaea*) grow and what does it look like, anyhow? It is evergreen, native to the Mediterranean region but grown in tropical areas and warm climates. The hard, yellow wood of the gnarled trunk is covered by gray-green bark. The branches extend to a height of 25 feet or more.

The leathery olive leaves are elliptic, oblong, or lanceolate in shape. They are dark green on top and have silvery scales underneath. The fragrant white flowers grow in axillary panicles that are shorter than the leaves. The fruit is an oblong or nearly round drupe that is shiny black when ripe. The best part is, the life span of an olive tree can be more than 1,500 years.

(*Source*: Olivus.)

OIL, GREEKS, AND ROMANS

The Greeks and Romans both share legends about olives and their creation by the gods. At the ancient Olympic Games, winners were awarded an olive tree branch. The Greeks believed that the life of the sacred tree was transmitted to the taker through the branch. Even more amazing, it's been said that the Greeks valued the golden liquid to such an extent that they allowed only virgin boys and girls to pick olives.[8]

In ancient Greece and Rome, olive oil was a respected commodity (as well as taxed) and carried by trading ships to all the Mediterranean countries. The concept that olive oil provides strength and youth made it a precious liquid to have and to hold. Aromatics (such as sage and rose) were added to olive oil to make ointments as well as fuel for lamps. In Greece, Rome, and Egypt, olive oil was infused with flowers and grasses to make both beauty aids and medicine.[9]

Therapeutic Oil Formula of the Four Thieves

In the Middle Ages, oil made its mark during the scourge of the bubonic plague, or "Black Death," of Europe. Robbers in the French town of Marseilles stole the belongings left behind by the people who fell victim to the outbreak.

The legend is that these robbers were spice traders and perfumers. To avoid the deadly plague, they put the magic of their essential oils (such as garlic, eucalyptus, lemon, rosemary, and sage) to work by washing themselves with the infection-fighting liquid. Later, the thieves' oil formula was used by priests and doctors who treated the ill.

The Roman Empire embraced the cultivation of olive groves. But when the Roman Empire fell, the olive groves died, although some trees continued to thrive in Tuscany. In A.D. 1100, olive groves sprouted again, and Tuscany became a well-known region for harvesting the olive tree. In fact, in 1400, Italy was ranked the number-one producer of olive oil on the globe.[10]

By the fifteenth century B.C., olive cultivation had extended from Crete, Greece, to Syria, Palestine, and Israel, and then to Turkey, Cyprus, and Egypt. Until 1500 B.C., it was in Greece, however, according to reports, where olive trees were most widespread. After the sixteenth century, olive trees were also found in Spain.[11]

In the eighteenth century, Franciscan missionaries carried the first olive trees to America. And then, in the nineteenth century, olive oil became a well-known commodity in the United States when Italian and Greek immigrants demanded the golden liquid to be imported from Europe. Once a European treasure, olive oil soon also became as good as gold to the chefs in the New World.[12]

OLIVE OIL MAKES A SPLASH IN AMERICA

In the 1950s (when I was born and raised surrounded by fruit orchards in San Jose, California), Ancel Keys, an American nutritionist and epidemiologist, conducted his famous Seven Countries Study. Keys and his colleagues studied the diet and health of the people in five European countries and compared their data with the data collected in similar studies in the United States and Japan. The findings: People who ate less saturated fat had lower levels of cholesterol and less heart disease than people who ate a high-saturated-fat diet.

During the 1950s, people, such as the Cretes in Greece, who followed a traditional Mediterranean diet and lifestyle—including using olive oil (a monounsaturated fat)—had lower cholesterol levels and lower rates of heart disease. It was believed that a diet chock-full of fresh vegetables, seasonal fruits, whole grains, fish, meats, and olive oil—like what was eaten in the Mediterranean basin—was a healthful, heart-healthy plan.

As time passed, in the 1950s and '60s, scientists started to study different types of fat—including polyunsaturated fats, which seemed to reduce cholesterol levels better than monounsaturated fats. This, in turn, resulted in praising Crisco (originated in the early twentieth century), corn oil, and margarine (oleo), which I remember sitting in our refrigerator along with plenty of frozen and processed foods, while shunning butter as a "bad" fat and calling olive oil "neutral."

Later, in the 1970s and '80s, when I was a vegan hippie and penniless graduate student, health-conscious people, like me, said so long to butter and margarine and began to use polyunsaturated vegetable oils in rice and vegetable dishes. At this time, I had no clue that researchers were busy at work labeling high-density lipoproteins (HDL) as "good" cholesterol and low-density lipoproteins (LDL) as "bad" cholesterol in our bodies. I was just a 20-something kid. What did I know?

Then, we were told that saturated fat raised the "bad" cholesterol and lowered the "good" cholesterol, but that vegetable oils (such as corn, safflower, soybean and margarine), while they lowered the "bad" LDL cholesterol, could also lower the "good" HDL cholesterol. So, dazed and confused, before I received my master's degree in May 1990, the word was out to use polyunsaturated vegetable fats sparingly, to stay clear of saturated animal fats, and to embrace monounsaturated fats like olive oil.

In 1990, when I was out of graduate school, the scientific jury was in. Research had shown that, rather than clog our arteries with saturated and polyunsaturated fats, we should turn to monounsaturated fats, which are rich in disease-fighting antioxidants.

Today, in the twenty-first century, olive oil (especially extra virgin olive oil) continues to gain praise worldwide for its vitamin E, phenol compounds, phytoestrogens, carotenoids, chlorophyll, and other good-for-you components. It plays a role in healthful cuisines—all types—in both restaurants and homes in the United States, as well as worldwide.

(*Source*: *The Flavors of Olive Oil* and a variety of other sources.)

OTHER PAST MEDICAL USES OF OLIVE OIL

Historical Olive Oil

User	Method	Ailment
Biblical priests	Olive oil paired with aromatics	To treat leprosy
Goddess Athena	Olive oil	To use as medicine
Greek athletes	Olive oil	To cleanse their bodies
Greeks, Egyptians, Romans	Infused olive tree flowers with grass or essential oils	To use as ointment for cuts, sores, bleeding wounds, bruises, and other injuries
Homer	Olive oil	Called it "liquid gold"
Hippocrates	Mixture of olive oil and leaves	To treat boils, cholera, inflammation of gums, muscle pain, nausea, and ulcers
Italians	Olive oil	To increase strength and youthful vitality
Christopher Columbus	Olive oil	Provided it to his exploring team

Sources: *The Passionate Olive, Healing Oils of the Bible,* and a wide variety of other books and Web sites.

OLIVE OIL MILESTONES

Year	What Happened	What It Did
1500s	Olive trees were part of the landscape in Spain	Spain ended up being the number-one olive oil producer
1600s	First olive press in the world was created on the island of Crete[13]	This paved the way for olive oil to be made and distributed
1800s	Olive oil made its debut in America	Olive oil was soon used by American cooks
1950s	Professor Ancel Keys, an American scientist, did research work to link the people of the Greek island of Crete to the Mediterranean diet	His Seven Countries Study showed that a diet low in saturated fat and high in monounsaturated and polyunsaturated fats may be the key to the Cretes' low rate of heart disease and increased longevity
1950s–1960s	Polyunsaturated fats were touted, saturated fats were shunned	This raised awareness about the dietary fat–health connection
1970s–1980s	HDL and LDL cholesterol was studied	"Bad" dietary fats such as polyunsaturated and saturated fats were linked to lowering "good" cholesterol and increasing "bad" cholesterol
1975	*How to Eat Well and Stay Well the Mediterranean Way* by Dr. Ancel Keys and Margaret Keys was published.	It popularized the heart-healthy diet

Year	What Happened	What It Did
1983	*Feast of the Olive* by Maggie Blythe Klein was published	It taught how to cook with olives and olive oil
1988	Anne Dolamore's *Essential Olive Oil Companion* was published	It allowed readers to appreciate not only the olive but also its oil
1980s	Consumers were told to use monounsaturated fats such as olive oil, to use small amounts of polyunsaturated fats, and to stay clear of saturated fats	This allowed people to lower their risk of heart disease by eating a heart-healthy diet
1990s	American scientists published articles on the Mediterranean diet	The articles linked lowered incidences of health problems with eating fresh vegetables, fruits, grains, fish, meats, and olive oil
1995	*Enter the Zone* by Barry Sears, Ph.D. was published	It praised "good" monounsaturated fats such as olive oil and olives
Early 2000s	Olive oil expands in popularity	Olive oil begins to play a role around the globe in diet, health, beauty, household use, and more

THE GOLDEN SECRETS TO REMEMBER

As you can see, "liquid gold" has been touted for centuries—in America and around the world—as a valuable healing medicine. Olive oil lovers past and present believe that healing oils—olive oil and other oils, too—add years to your life by:

✓ Acting as a medicinal agent—solo or teamed with herbs—to fight dozens of health ailments and diseases
✓ Fighting the infection of wounds
✓ Soothing inflammation, muscle pain, and other medical disorders
✓ Providing a versatile staple in meals
✓ Offering a symbol of peace worldwide
✓ Enhancing energy and stamina
✓ Acting as a heart-healthy food in the Mediterranean diet

No doubt, olive oil, since biblical times, has had an amazing track record of powerful health benefits. And it's continued to hold up its good name, as well as create a mighty buzz around the world. In Part 2, "Olive Oil," you'll discover some amazing facts and meet intriguing people from the Mediterranean world. Now it's time to get the lowdown on one of the world's most popular kinds of oil—olive oil—in the twentieth and twenty-first centuries.

PART 2

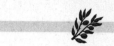

OLIVE OIL

A Historical Testimony

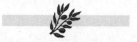

*Wash him in the stream of the river, Anoint him
with immortal oil, Put him on the divine tunic.*
—Homer[1]

Olive oil was healthy in the twentieth century, and it is healthy in the twenty-first century, too. While its uses are infinite—both inside and outside the body—its healing powers are due to its healthful ingredients. And now, research shows promising benefits of the nutrients in olive oil (which may be missing from our daily food intake thanks to processed foods) more than ever before. But these new findings would not be surprising to the folks who have touted olive oil through the decades.

OLIVE OIL PIONEERS IN THE TWENTIETH CENTURY

Born in 1915, Joseph Sciabica has been an olive oil maker since 1936. His father, Nicola, and he began with the grassroots of olive oil production, which he learned in Sicily, Italy, as a young man.

In Waterbury, Connecticut, in the 1940s, it was common for Joseph to deliver a load of wine grapes and olive oil to an Italian family in the city. In fact, Nick Sciabica & Sons sold olive oil directly to Italian families from 1936 to 1968.

Today, in his nineties, Joseph, who has resided in Modesto, California, for 63 years, has 40 acres with 1,000 olive trees. He and his wife, Gemma, have passed their knowledge on to both their sons, Daniel and Nick, and their grandson Jonathan. These days, Nick Sciabica & Sons makes 100 percent extra virgin natural cold-pressed olive oil.

Gemma Sanita Sciabica, a charming Italian woman in her eighties, also from Connecticut, has been married to Joseph for 63 years. She is a nutrition-savvy cook who has been creating healthful Italian-based recipes for years. Her cookbooks, such as *Cooking with California Olive Oil: Treasured Family Recipes*, are filled with heart-healthy recipes from the old Mediterranean world. But there are other olive growers in California, too, who have helped spread the healthful oil worldwide.

In the 1990s, once olive oil was embraced by America for its health benefits, California jumped on the Mediterranean bandwagon. "Wineries in Napa and Sonoma began to plant a few olives as an adjunct to their main business. The first grower to import Italian olives was Ridgely Evers of Healdsburg in 1990. He was followed by Nan McEvoy and Roberto Zecca, owners of Frantoio Restaurant," writes Charles Quest-Ritson in his book *Olive Oil* (DK Publishing, 2006).[2]

While I did not get to meet Zecca face to face, I did talk with him briefly on the telephone. Better still, I visited his unique and impressive restaurant. I knew, however, that Zecca has a place in the olive oil world, both in Italy and in Mill Valley, California.

As the story goes, in 1989, the retired banker and his wife, Christina, decided to relocate to the hills of Greve in Chianti. They bought a *Castellare*, which is a castle-villa. They began to make extra virgin olive oil from the grove of olive trees surrounding their home. At first, they made the healthy oil for their personal use, and then they began to sell it to local markets.[3]

A few years later, the couple came to Northern California and opened a one-of-a-kind restaurant that included a *frantoio*, or olive press.[4] In the fall of 1995, the Frantoio Olive Oil Co. produced its first crush. And these days, Zecca offers an olive oil tagged Select Sevillano, as well as provides a popular place to enjoy great Italian cuisine and view the making of healthy extra virgin olive oil.

A Toast to the Green Olive and Martini

Before California olive oil pioneers made their mark in the Golden State, another pioneer, of sorts, brought the world the green olive in a dry martini. I prefer the story linking the concoction to a gold miner in Martinez, in Northern California. Back in the mid-nineteenth century, the miner understandably wanted to celebrate his gold strike. At a bar, he asked for a special drink made with gin and vermouth and topped with bitters and a maraschino cherry. The drink was coined the "martini," in respect of the town Martinez. Decades later, someone else opted to use a green olive instead of a cherry. And today, some people use different garnishes, from a slice of lemon peel to two green olives.

MR. CHOLESTEROL—DR. ANCEL KEYS

Ancel Keys, Ph.D., who was born in 1904 and lived nearly 100 years, is the man who focused on one of America's biggest problems, past and present—heart disease. He is the genius behind the Seven Countries Study. For several decades, he kept his eyes on 12,000 middle-aged men from Italy, the Greek Islands, Yugoslavia, the Netherlands, Finland, Japan, and the United States. His findings were that saturated fat (found in butter and cheese) was linked to high cholesterol and heart attacks.

However, a Mediterranean diet based on fresh vegetables, fruit, bread, pasta—and the monounsaturated fat olive oil—showed that low cholesterol and heart attacks were not part of the picture. He made the diet–heart disease connection. In fact, in the 1950s, when Keys visited Greece to find out why Cretes lived longer than the people of other cultures, he was astonished by how much olive oil these people used on their salads.

Dr. Keys is known for two diets he popularized. He created balanced meals for soldiers that were called "K rations." Later on, the health-conscious doctor and his wife, Margaret, made the Mediterranean diet known through two books, *Eat Well and Stay Well* (Doubleday, 1959) and *How to Eat Well and Stay Well the Mediterranean Way* (Doubleday, 1975).

OLIVE OYL LINKS TO OIL

In the 1950s and '60s, while serious doctors were praising the powers of olive oil, kids and their parents watched the popular *Popeye* cartoons, which also were linked to olive oil, but in a humorous way that made its impression on a large audience, too.

Elzie Segar created Olive Oyl for his comic strip, "Thimble Theater," back in 1919. The tall, thin cartoon character with black hair is named after olive oil. Segar's newspaper comics also feature a variety of Olive Oyl's relatives, tagged after other oils, such as her brother, Castor Oyl, and their mother, Nan Oyl (after banana oil).[5]

Olive Oyl gained popularity in the animated television cartoons, where she is Popeye's girlfriend. Bluto (also known as the bully Brutus) is Popeye's competition for Olive's attention, but the sailor always eats his spinach and rescues the damsel in distress, who ironically has a baby named Swee' Pea.

CONTEMPORARY DOCTORS: THE OLIVE OIL ADVOCATES

In 1996, I interviewed best-selling author Dr. Barry Sears, who had written the popular book *Enter the Zone* (HarperCollins, 1995). Working on a weight-loss-diet story for *Woman's World* magazine, I was a bit surprised when the doctor told me fat was part of his dietary plan, since I was writing about low-fat and fat-free foods. But today, I understand that he was ahead of his time.

More than 10 years ago, he wrote in his book that while saturated fats should be kept to a minimum, there are also "good" fats. He put it this way: "Most of the good fats are monounsaturated fats—those found in olive oil, canola oil, olives, macadamia nuts, and avocados (and, of course, guacamole). (A diet rich in monounsaturated fats is sometimes called a Mediterranean diet.)"

In a nutshell, he advised staying clear of "bad" fats such as saturated fats (found in animal protein sources and whole-fat dairy products), and get most of your daily fat from "good," monounsaturated fat.

While the Zone diet is a high-protein diet, Dr. Sears is still an advocate of "good" fats rich in monounsaturated fat.

On the flip side, Jan McBarron, M.D., a Columbus, Georgia, weight-loss specialist, has put protein on the side. She includes olive oil (like Dr. Sears recommends), but she shed unwanted pounds herself by following a Mediterranean-type diet and lifestyle. She eats heartily early in the day, focuses on complex carbohydrates, keeps protein intake moderate, has small snacks throughout the day, and gets moderate exercise.

Dr. McBarron's meal plan is based on complex carbohydrates. A diet of 70 percent complex carbs—vegetables, fruits, pasta, rice, bread, lentils, peas, and beans—provides more energy than one full of protein-rich foods, so you'll burn more fat, she says. "Complex carbohydrates also stimulate the production of serotonin, a brain chemical that can ease stress that leads to overeating." And speaking of food . . .

Dr. McBarron adds, "I'm married to an Italian. He grew up having pasta seven days a week. We always have pasta on the table. I'll have it four to five times a week. My husband is extremely healthy. He was raised on a healthy diet. When I met him I always did the salad dressing on the side because I was trying to watch my weight. And he always had oil and vinegar. I thought, 'Oh, that sounds terrible.' I don't even have salad dressing in my house anymore—it's always oil and vinegar for the taste and nutrients in it." And olive oil is more than a good-for-you food. It's a sacred oil to some people.

OLIVE OIL IN RELIGION

Before I take you back into the world of nutrition and your kitchen, I can't ignore the fact that olive oil is dished up in religion and folk magic. It is common knowledge that olive oil has been used for centuries by Christians as well as the ancient Hebrews. The sacred oil was also used for anointing the kings of the Kingdom of Israel and in religious ceremonies of the ancient Minoans.

"During baptism in the Christian church, holy oil, which is often olive oil, may be used for anointment. At the Chrism mass olive oil blessed by the bishop, 'chrism,' is used in the ceremony," explains John Deane, M.D.

As a Catholic woman, religion and holy oil brings back fond childhood memories of learning the seven sacraments and playing a role in some of them—which included using olive oil. In fact, before 1970, olive oil was used in four of the seven sacraments—Baptism, Confirmation, Holy Orders, and Anointing of the Sick. In 1970, holy oils were allowed to come from any plant, not just olives. But olive oil is still used in most dioceses, and the only reason it is not used is that it isn't available.

Baptism: I know firsthand that the Catholic and Orthodox Churches use olive oil for the Oil of Catechumen (used to bless and strengthen those preparing for Baptism). At Saint Joseph's Church in San Jose, California, I was baptized on the sixteenth of November 1952 according to the Rite of the Roman Catholic Church. At 10 days old, I had the sign of the cross made on my forehead with the holy oil.

Anointing of the Sick: I recall when I was 10 years old, our neighbor, Dale, was suffering with many illnesses. She was wheelchair-bound and in pain from the effects of polio. She, like my family, was Catholic. My mom told me that a priest from our parish paid her a home visit to bless her. These days, I know that this sacrament is called "Anointing of the Sick." Again, the blessed olive oil was used in a sign of the cross on both her forehead and hands.

Confirmation: As a teenager, I was confirmed at Saint Frances Cabrini's Church in San Jose, California. My confirmation name was Theresa, chosen by me. Again, I was anointed by a bishop who used the sign of the cross on my forehead during the ceremony. Today, I still feel bonded to the Catholic Church. However, I am open-minded and don't judge other religions.

PRACTICAL MAGIC

A few years ago, *Complete Woman* magazine asked me to write a few articles on Wiccans, or witches. At that time, the film *Practical Magic,* with Sandra Bullock and Nicole Kidman, was hot. Also, the TV program *Charmed* was "in," and everyone had loved the TV sitcom *Bewitched,* which ended up as a film.

So, while countless people believe magic is evil, I learned that the days of witch hunts are over. The image of an old hag riding her broomstick on a moonlit night is fading. New generations of good witches who do a little practical magic (using natural ingredients such as olive oil!) are sweeping the world with their feminine witchery (there are male wizards, too) and, of course, their wonderful cats.

Welcome to today's witch. An estimated 3 million witches live in the United States today. The word "witch" is derived from *Wicce*, an Anglo-Saxon word meaning "wise one." Today, men and women are gaining personal empowerment through a matriarchal, nature-based religion called Wicca. Wiccans are often young, college-educated, and middle-class, and many of them have families and cats. (Refer to the popular TV program *Charmed*.)

If you check out some Web sites touting folk magic or Wicca, you will quickly find many spells and potions that include natural ingredients from Mother Nature—olive oil and essential oils are included. Also, I recall from the articles I wrote about Wiccans that they can and do cast good spells for a variety of good reasons and occasions.

The Get Well Spell

"This spell uses olive oil as the focus of the spell. Olive oil has been used for centuries as a sacred oil, and was burned at churches and during ancient rituals. Ruled by the Sun and by the element of fire, it imparts strength to overcome all obstacles," explains Dark Raven, a self-proclaimed Wiccan of North Carolina.

Here, take a close-up look at Dark Raven's original three-day healing spell, to be used in preparing for surgery or recovering from a major health ailment or disease. You can cast it for yourself, a family member, a friend, or even a companion animal.

Tools:
One 6-inch red taper candle (and candleholder)
Rosemary
Bay leaves (whole or crushed)
Olive oil
Picture of the person who is ill (or the person's name written on a piece of paper)
Altar pentacle
Mortar and pestle
Incense burner with charcoal
Cauldron or other fire-safe container

Timing: Waxing moon (when the moon disk is growing). This is a three-day spell, so be sure to cast it in a place where your tools can remain undisturbed for three days.

Preparation: Add the rosemary and bay leaves to your mortar. Add a few drops of olive oil and crush the ingredients together to create an oily incense (slightly oily—not dripping with oil). Take your candle and make two marks on it to divide it into three equal parts. If you wish, scribe the name of the person or a rune of strength and healing on each part of the candle. Make sure you get the permission of the sick person if you are casting the spell for someone else. If you do not have a picture of the sick person, write the person's name on a piece of paper.

Casting the Spell:

Can an olive oil spell work magic? It's worth a try if healing is on your mind.

Day One: Cast your circle. Light your charcoal and drop your incense on it; be sure to keep your incense burning during the entire spell. Place the picture of the person (or his or her name on a piece of paper) at the center of your altar pentacle. Form an image of the person in your mind, imagine the person healthy and happy, but think of only the person—not of his or her illness. Anoint the candle with olive oil. As you do, continue to think of the person, using the oil as a medium to infuse the candle with your image of the person. Place the candle in the candleholder and place the candleholder in the center of your altar pentacle, over the picture of the person (or the piece of paper with his or her name). Light the candle. Watch the flame and feel the strength the fire brings. Imagine that strength traveling to the person. Meditate on how that person will be strong and will use this strength to overcome all illness. Picture the person happy and strong and doing the things that he or she enjoys doing. Focus and meditate on this until the candle burns down to the first mark. Snuff out the candle, and leave your spell area undisturbed.

Day Two: Cast your circle. Light your charcoal and drop your incense on it; be sure to keep your incense burning during the entire spell. Light the candle. Watch the flame and feel the strength the fire brings. Imagine that strength traveling to the ill person. Meditate on how that person will be strong and will use this strength to overcome all illness. Picture the person happy and strong and doing the things that he or she enjoys doing. Focus and meditate on this until the candle burns down to the second mark. Snuff out the candle, and leave your spell area undisturbed.

Day Three: Cast your circle. Light your charcoal and drop your incense on it; be sure to keep your incense burning during the entire spell. Light the candle. Watch the flame and feel the strength the fire brings. Imagine that strength traveling to the ill person. Meditate on how that person will be strong and will use this strength to overcome all illness. Picture the person happy and strong and doing the things that he or she enjoys doing. Focus and meditate on this until the candle burns down almost completely. When the candle is almost burned down, take the picture of the person or the piece of paper with his or her name, and light it with the flame of the candle. Let the picture burn up in your cauldron or other fire-safe container. Let the candle burn all the way down. Feel the strength that you have sent the person. Finish your spell by saying, "This is my will, so mote it be!"

Bright Blessings,
Dark Raven
www.ravenmoonlight.com

These days, while people use olive oil for religion, food, medicine, cosmetics, home cures, and lamps, there is an enormous supply of sturdy olive trees. But I have discovered that nobody knows for sure how many olive trees exist on Earth. According to the North American Olive Oil Association, there are now more than 800 million olive trees planted worldwide. Paul Vossen of the University of California Co-operative Extension in Sonoma County, who studies the olive oil industry and educates its farmers, told me there are more than 24 million acres full of olive trees around the globe. The number of olive varieties, he adds, is around 2,500 to 3,000.

While people are putting olive oil to work in a variety of ways, there are also a number of powerful components that deserve due credit. In the next chapter, I'll show you what research has revealed about olive oil and its supernutrients—which are missing more and more from the diet here in America, in the Mediterranean basin, and worldwide.

THE GOLDEN SECRETS TO REMEMBER

✓ Extra virgin olive oil, which is polyphenol-rich, was made and sold in the early 1900s by olive oil pioneers on the East Coast who helped bring this liquid gold to the West Coast of America.

✓ Olive "oyl" and spinach—two healthy foods—were introduced in the early twentieth century in cartoons; and in the nineteenth century, the green olive made its debut in a popular alcoholic mixed drink.

✓ Olive oil has been used in religion for centuries—and in the twentieth century, the blessed oil was used as the main ingredient in four sacraments of the Catholic religion, and in other religions, too.

✓ Mother Nature's natural resources such as oil—including olive oil—are used in healthful spells and potions by witches and Wiccans to help heal themselves and people who come to them for healing.

Where Are the Secret Ingredients?

*The grape and the olive are among the priceless
benefactions of the soil, and were destined, each in
its way, to promote the welfare of man.*
—George Ellwanger[1]

I remember what it was like when I hitched and hiked through
America in the winter of 1974 with a knapsack and a Labrador Retriever.
There we were, on our own and it was up to me to feed us a healthful
diet.

In the Midwest, I admit to snacking on candy bars, diet soda, and
processed snacks. But in the Northeast on my way to Quebec, Canada,
I did go on a health kick. I packed the essentials such as whole grain
bread, peanut butter, dried fruit, and nuts. But at truck stops, I remember using salad dressings on salads and resorting to table scraps
for my dog. I didn't use olive oil on vegetables nor did I carry it with
me.

Although we weathered a blizzard, a sandstorm, desert heat and a
monsoon season, I wonder, what if we had eaten a more balanced diet
and included olive oil with its wealth of good ingredients? No matter,
we both had youth, plenty of exercise and the great outdoors on our

side. But if I had to do it all over again, I would have carried extra virgin olive oil in my pack. Here's why.

When you look at extra virgin olive oil's product label, it appears to be a health-minded person's ideal food: no trans fats, cholesterol, or sodium. But when I read the nutrition label, I didn't see vitamins or minerals. So, where are the powerful nutrients in olive oil, anyhow?

Nutrition Facts
Serving Size 1 Tablespoon (14 g)
Amount per serving

Calories 120	
Calories from fat 120	
Trans Fat 0 g	
Polyunsaturated Fat 1 g	
Monounsaturated Fat 11 g	
Cholesterol 0 mg	
Sodium 0 mg	
Total Carbohydrate 0 g	
Protein 0 g	

Source: Spectrum Naturals.

Dazed and confused, I went straight to the olive oil experts at the Olive Oil Council and obtained a nutritional breakdown of the golden liquid. The nutrition facts seem to be a bit different, and the measurements a bit bigger.

Supersize Olive Oil, Anyone?

100 grams (3½ ounces) of olive oil contains:

100 percent fat
1 milligram calcium
0.56 milligram iron
1 milligram potassium
2 milligrams sodium
0.3 milligram choline

0.1 milligram betaine
14.35 milligrams vitamin E
60.2 micrograms vitamin K
13.808 grams fatty acids, total saturated
72.961 grams fatty acids, total monounsaturated
10.523 fatty acids, total polyunsaturated
221 milligrams phytosterols

Apparently, more olive oil equals more nutrients. One cup contains about two times the amount of fat, calories, vitamins, and minerals.

(*Source:* National Nutrient Database for Standard Reference, 2006.)

People who have written about olive oil claim that olive oil is chock-full of nutrients, minerals, and vitamins. True, the golden liquid does contain essential nutrients if you drink the stuff. The bottom line: Researchers know that quality extra virgin olive oil contains disease-fighting polyphenols, as well as other nutrients that can be effective if teamed with the Mediterranean diet and lifestyle. In other words, it's not the olive oil by itself that can contain healing powers. Speaking of olive oil . . .

QUALITY COUNTS

Not all olive oil is nutrient-rich, natural, organic, extra virgin olive oil made using the cold-pressed method. Some producers slow down the process or use heat so that the oil will taste better and can be preserved longer.

The fact is, the best olive oils are made from polyphenol-rich olives and cold-pressed within 24 to 48 hours after harvesting. This is the ideal way.

Olive oil contains the same important nutrients as olives—fat, calcium, and vitamins E and K—plus it contains other nutritional components.

So, What's in an Olive, Anyhow?

Three-and-one-half ounces of olives contains:

163 calories
70.8 percent water
1.2 grams protein
18.6 grams fat
1.7 grams fiber
79 milligrams calcium
200 international units vitamin A
0.01 milligram vitamin B_1
0.18 milligram vitamin B_2
0.1 milligram vitamin B_3
3 milligrams vitamin C
2.3 international units vitamin E

(*Source:* John Deane, M.D.)

SIX SUPER HEALTH-PROMOTING OLIVE OIL COMPONENTS

1 **Essential Fatty Acids:** Oleic acid is monounsaturated and makes up 55 to 85 percent of olive oil. Linoleic is polyunsaturated and makes up about 9 percent. Linolenic, which is polyunsaturated, makes up 0 to 1.5 percent. These types of fats, unlike saturated and trans fats, are heart healthy and much more.

Olive oil has no trans fatty acid. That's right; it has no unhealthy artery-clogging trans fats. It isn't a trans fatty acid because it hasn't been partially hydrogenated in a factory to make it solid at room temperature, like margarine.

Both omega-3 and omega-6 fatty acids also are in olive oil. Omega-3 fatty acids are important in preventing heart disease and are high in oily fish, such as salmon, and flaxseed oil. The jury is still out about how much omega-3 versus omega-6 you should incorporate into your daily diet.

Foods rich in essential fatty acids include fish, olive oils, fish oils and flaxseed oils. Team the olive oil with fish in our Simple Salmon dish, and you'll get both "good" fats and good taste, too.

2 **Antioxidants:** Like essential fatty acids, the polyphenols in olive oil are good for your body from head to toe. Natural antioxidants have been scientifically proven to have a variety of health benefits, from healing sunburn to lowering cholesterol, blood pressure, and the risk of heart disease. There are as many as 5 milligrams of antioxidant polyphenols in every 10 grams of olive oil, according to Dr. Deane.

Vitamin E, for one, is a natural antioxidant in olive oil. One tablespoon provides 8 percent of the RDA for vitamin E. Research shows that people who eat antioxidant-rich foods such as vegetable oils, fruits, vegetables, grains, and nuts lower their risk of getting heart disease and cancer.

You can get antioxidants by eating antioxidant-rich foods such as vegetables and vitamin-E-rich olive oil. Just whip up a batch of our Sesame-Almond Vegetable Sauté, and enjoy.

3 **Calcium:** Olive oil also contains a trace of needed calcium. If your diet is deficient in calcium, your body will steal it from your bones. This, in turn, will weaken your skeleton and can lead to brittle bone disease.

Note these other important calcium facts:

- Ninety percent of the body's calcium is stored in the bones and teeth.
- One percent is found in the blood and tissues.
- Calcium is necessary for transmitting nerve impulses and regulating muscle contraction.
- The need for calcium starts in infancy and continues throughout life.

While olive oil may contain only a small amount of bone-boosting calcium, you can add it to calcium-rich dishes. Also, you don't have to stick with milk, yogurt, or cheese. Calcium is found in broccoli, green leafy vegetables, and tofu. Try our Summer Vegetable and Organic Tofu Tacos for that calcium fix you need.

4 **Iron:** Not only does your body need calcium, but it requires iron, too. As with calcium, olive oil contains just a small amount of iron, but you can certainly use it to make iron-rich dishes taste

better. No, liver isn't the only source of iron. Remember Popeye? He got his iron from spinach. Go ahead—give our Seared Boneless Breast of Chicken Stuffed with Spinach and Basil a try, and don't forget Olive "Oyl"—a must-have companion.

5 **Potassium:** Olive oil, again, contains just a small amount of potassium. But don't forget that olive oil can be teamed with vegetables, and that is where you're going to get plenty of potassium. It's the potassium that helps energize you. Low potassium levels bring on fatigue. Often, people who suffer from nutritional deficiencies (due to anorexia, fad diets, or alcoholism) lack enough potassium. You need a daily minimum of 1,875 milligrams of potassium, and healthful extra virgin olive oil used in vegetable salads and stir-fries can help you get that. Take a peek at our Panzanella (Tuscan Tomato & Bread Salad) and enjoy. Keep in mind, one cup of canned tomatoes contains 500 to 750 milligrams of potassium.

6 **Vitamin K:** Olive oil does contain a sufficient amount of this vitamin, which is important for bone formation because it binds calcium to the bone matrix. You need 70 to 140 micrograms of vitamin K each day. The best sources are spinach, parsley, and turnips. To get that dose of this bone-boosting vitamin, enjoy a spinach salad drizzled with olive oil.

OTHER OLIVE OIL INGREDIENTS

Aromatic substances: These are what give olive oil its taste and smell.
Coloring substances: These include carotenoids and chlorophyll, both of which have disease-fighting antioxidant benefits.
Hydrocarbons: These may be good for cholesterol, and their beta-carotene content has both vitamin A and antioxidant benefits.
Phytoestrogens: These may help beat bone loss as well as lessen hot flashes. In some Asian countries, where women consume plenty of phytoestrogen-rich soy, hot flashes are not common. (A bonus: Team soy with olive oil. I sailed though minor menopausal hot flashes by taking soy supplements.)

If you want to enhance your diet with photoestrogens, use olive oil, an edible phytoestrogen, with other foods that contain phytoestrogens, such as apples, asparagus, beans, blackberries, carrots, cherries, corn, flaxseed, garlic, green pepper, oat bran, onions, pears, squash, sunflower seeds, wheat germ, and yams. And yes, many of the heart-healthy recipes in this book include these foods.

Sterols: These may inhibit the absorption of dietary cholesterol.

Olive Oil Health Boosters

What It Is and Does	May Help Prevent
VITAMIN E: slows down the aging of skin and hair cells; helps to repair damaged muscle in the back; decreases free-radical damage.	Cancer (stomach, lung, larynx, esophagus), Parkinson's disease
VITAMIN K: reduces calcium and bone loss.	Osteoporosis
CALCIUM: maintains strong, healthy bones and teeth, which store 99 percent of the body's calcium; assists enzymes in fat and protein digestion and energy production; helps regulate the contraction of muscles, including the heart; aids the absorption of other nutrients.	Osteoporosis
IRON: plays a role in immune system functioning and is important to cognition.	Anemia
OMEGA-3s AND 6s: important for the lubrication of the joints; can serve as precursors for anti-inflammatory substances in the body such as prostaglandins (inflammation is one of the problems that contribute to asthma).	Heart disease, arthritis, inflammatory bowel disease, diabetes

What It Is and Does	May Help Prevent
POTASSIUM: plays a role in regulating blood pressure; balances out sodium levels to prevent water retention.	High blood pressure, heart disease, stroke, obesity

So, teaming olive oil with nutrient-rich foods is the way to go to enhance your total health. But how exactly does this liquid, once considered as good as gold, help your body to keep the doctor away and stave off disease? Scientists, medical doctors, nutritionists, and everyday people will show you how olive oil can be your best food friend—with no strings attached.

THE GOLDEN SECRETS TO REMEMBER

✓ Olive oil contains plenty of healthful nutrients.

✓ The quality of olive oil counts. Natural, organic, and made using the fast cold-pressed method is recommended by olive oil producers and medical doctors.

✓ Olives, from which olive oil is made, contain a variety of nutrients, including fiber, calcium, and vitamins A, C, and E.

✓ Essential fatty acids, the miracle workers of olive oil, help prevent heart disease and a variety of other diseases and health ailments.

✓ Olive oil contains antioxidants, calcium, iron, potassium, and vitamin K.

✓ Other good stuff, such as phytoestrogens and sterols, is also found in olive oil.

✓ The total ingredients of olive oil—especially when the oil is paired with a nutritious diet—can help prevent pesky health ailments and stave off life-threatening diseases.

Why Is Olive Oil So Healthy?

*Olive oil is the best and safest of all oils. It tastes
good, too.*

—Andrew Weil, M.D.[1]

In college, I was a nanny, of sorts, for affluent families in the San
Francisco Bay Area. One luxury home in Los Gatos stands out in my
mind. It was owned by a medical doctor and his beautiful Italian wife,
complete with three kids who lived in amid Mediterranean décor that
I cherished.

In the kitchen, there was always fresh fruit and vegetables somewhere in sight. In fact, the doctor's wife always sent me home with a
treat, whether it was guavas or lemons from their fruit trees in the
front yard. And yes, there was the lingering aroma of garlic, and onions
sizzling in olive oil in a large pan with a special dinner in the making.

I always felt a liveliness and feel-good vibe when I did my chores as
I smelled the scent of good food throughout the house. And these
days, I maintain that type of ambience in my own Tuscan-style kitchen
(i.e., family-style wooden table, colorful Italian pottery, iron candle
holders and hues of golds and reds) with something olive oil-based
baking or cooking and fresh fruit and vegetables out on the counter-
tops. It helps feed the body, mind, and spirit. What's more, there is
proof that olive oil—the important food—is healthy.

Do you know that stacks and stacks of studies show that polyphenol-rich extra virgin olive oil can and does help to lower the risk of developing health ailments and diseases (at any age)? Here's a look at some research that you can put to work in your life to stay healthier.

8 HEALTH VIRTUES OF OLIVE OIL

1 **Cuts Risk of Heart Disease** For thousands of years, people around the Mediterranean Sea, including the residents of the Holy Land, have had lower rates of heart disease. The consensus is that olive oil is the common thread.

How Olive Oil Works: Studies show that a daily intake of olive oil lowers the risk of heart disease of all kinds, including heart attack. Olive oil has been shown to thin the blood, lower the blood pressure, and regulate cholesterol by reducing the "bad" kind (LDL) while maintaining the "good" kind (HDL). A healthful diet and lifestyle are key weapons in the battle to prevent heart disease—America's number-one killer for both men and women, according to the American Heart Association (AHA).

The good news is that olive oil may come to the rescue in America as it has for centuries in the Mediterranean world. Virgin olive oil may be more heart healthy than other vegetable fats, according to new research. European scientists have discovered virgin olive oil may help lower heart disease risk because of its high level of antioxidant plant compounds, according to a study published in the *Annals of Internal Medicine.*[2]

In a study of 200 young and middle-aged healthy men, three olive oils were used for three weeks. One oil was a virgin olive oil rich in poylphenols. The other two were processed with moderate to low polyphenols. The findings: The researchers discovered that polyphenol-rich virgin olive oil showed stronger heart-health effects than the more processed "non-virgin" types. Virgin olive oil is more than just a heart-healthy monounsaturated fat. Polyphenols, claim the authors, may be the key to some of the health benefits linked to this healing oil. The scientific jury is still out, however, before the researchers recommend virgin olive oil as a replacement for other vegetable oils.

What You Can Do: Both polyunsaturated fats (safflower, sesame seeds, soybeans, many nuts and seeds, and their oils) and monounsaturated fats (canola, olive, and peanut oils, and avocado) may help to lower your blood cholesterol and blood pressure when you use them in place of saturated fats in your diet, reports the AHA. (See Chapter 10, "The Elixir to Heart Health," for more studies and recommendations to lower your risk of heart attack and stroke, beat high blood pressure and cholesterol, and prevent or control diabetes.)

2 **Fights Cancer** While heart disease goes back to biblical times, cancer probably does, too. "Because of its aromatic oil content, olive oil is an effective antioxidant that has been shown to reduce cancer rates and increase longevity," points out *Healing Oils of the Bible*'s author, Dr. Stewart.[3]

How Olive Oil Works: Researchers at Copenhagen University Hospital in Denmark discovered that olive oil can reduce damage to cells, which can trigger cancer growth. For three weeks, 182 healthy men between the ages of 20 and 60 from five European countries consumed about one-fourth cup of olive oil every day. The findings: There was a 13 percent reduction in a marker of damage to cells. It's the phenols, believed to act as powerful disease-fighting antioxidants. In addition, the results (published in *The Federation of American Societies for Experimental Biology Journal*) may point to why the cancer rate is higher in northern Europe than in southern Europe, where olive oil is part of the olive-rich Mediterranean diet.[4]

Oleic acid, the main monounsaturated fatty acid in olive oil, as well as disease-fighting phenols may be the two primary components that lower the risk of developing skin, breast, and colon cancer.[5]

What You Can Do: The American Cancer Society (ACS) advises that you eat five to nine servings of fruits and vegetables daily to help lower your risk of developing cancer. Polyphenol-rich olive oil can help enhance the flavor of fresh produce, but the ACS does not validate olive oil used solo as a preventive measure for lowering the risk of developing cancer. But the ACS does note that lycopene, found in tomato products, does help in the prevention of some cancers, such as prostate cancer. Go ahead— enjoy vegetarian pizza or pasta with tomato sauce, because the effects of lycopene are increased when lycopene-rich vegetables are cooked and eaten together with fat.

3 **Wards Off Arthritis** Not only are there lower rates of cancer in the Mediterranean basin than in other countries, research in Greece also showed that the more fresh vegetables and olive oil people ate, the less likely they were to develop rheumatoid arthritis. Also, it's possible that the omega-3-rich fish eaten in a typical Greek diet may play a role in keeping stiffness, aches, and pains away, too.

Olive oil combined externally with soothing essential oils, which soothe muscle aches and pains, may have beneficial effects for arthritis aches and pains, often an age-related disease that can be worse in cold, damp climates. When I dined at Frantoio's, a staff member told me without hesitation that a regular customer vows that it's the extra virgin olive oil in his diet that keeps his arthritis at bay. I believed him.

How Olive Oil Works: Olive oil used daily may have anti-inflammatory benefits for pain by lubricating joints and reducing swelling. Also, folk doctors believe eating cooked antioxidant-rich vegetables with olive oil provides polyunsaturated and mono-unsaturated fats that are used by your body to make the good prostaglandins that reduce swelling and pain.

What You Can Do: Include olive oil in your daily diet. While some folks use olive oil on their salads and cooked vegetables and eat fish to help stave off arthritis, others turn to olive oil paired with essential oils in massages to loosen up stiff muscles and joints.

4 **Keeps Diabetes at Bay** Diabetes (type 2), like arthritis, has been a problem for a long time. Worse, the numbers are soaring for both baby boomers and senior citizens. We can blame high blood sugar on a high-fat diet, excess weight, and a sedentary lifestyle.

How Olive Oil Works: It's believed that olive oil can cut the amount of "bad" LDL cholesterol as well as triglycerides, also known as fats, in your blood. This, in turn, may help to lower your risk of developing type 2 diabetes, which can be controlled by making diet and lifestyle changes. Olive oil may also lower your blood sugar. Why? The good effect may be due to olive oil being a monounsaturated fat.

What You Can Do: Eat a low-fat, heart-healthy "fishatarian" diet, which is plant-based, low in fat, and full of whole grains, legumes, fruits, and vegetables. Keep your weight in check, and do not overdo your intake of olive oil, since a high-fat diet can lead to weight gain and other health problems.

5 **Stops Pain** Diabetes is often painless, especially before it gets out of control, but pain can be a pain in the rear. "Olive oil has also been used as a healing ointment for centuries by Greeks, Romans, Egyptians, Christians, and Jews. While usually combined with essential oils, it was routinely applied to cuts, sores, bleeding wounds, bruises, and injuries of all kinds, with a little wine as antiseptic," notes Dr. Stewart.[6]

How Olive Oil Works: Research shows that olive oil contains a chemical, oleocanthal, that can stop inflammation similar to painkillers such as ibuprofen and other anti-inflammatory medications.

What You Can Do: Use olive oil topically to help heal cuts, sores, and other ailments that involve inflammation, redness, and pain. Also, it couldn't hurt to include olive oil in your daily diet as well, since it may help to strengthen your immune system and speed up the healing process. Plus, we know that omega-3s can help reduce inflammation, which often creates pain.

6 **Inhibits Loss of Memory** While none of us wants to be in physical pain, mental illness can be a nightmare, too. Alzheimer's is a brain disease that affects brain function. Its symptoms include tearjerker film–like loss of independence and relationship woes, as depicted in *On Golden Pond* and *The Notebook,* in which char-

acters are trapped in their bodies as their minds and memories deteriorate.

How Olive Oil Works: Researchers at Columbia University Medical Center in New York studied about 2,000 adults (in their mid-seventies) including 194 who had Alzheimer's disease. They studied what the people ate in the year prior to the onset of the disease. The findings were that the closer a person's eating habits were to the Mediterranean diet, the lower his or her odds were of having Alzheimer's. The diet may help reduce brain inflammation and oxidation in the body. The monounsaturated acids are believed to maintain cell structure and membranes in the brain.[7]

What You Can Do: Include olive oil, an important monounsaturated fat source, in a Mediterranean-type diet.

7 **Beats Bone Loss** Losing your mind can be a challenge, but bone loss can be debilitating as well. The connection between bone density and fracture was made back in the late eighteenth century by Ashley Cooper, who coined the term "osteoporosis," once considered an old woman's problem.

How Olive Oil Works: The main polyphenol in olive oil, oleuropein, may prevent bone loss with inflammation. Olive oil is also believed to assist calcium absorption and to help beat bone loss and even reverse the crippling effects of osteoporosis. If your diet is deficient in calcium, your body will steal it from your bones. This will weaken your skeleton and can lead to the brittle bone disease. Fats such as olive oil are needed for proper calcium metabolism and are essential components of cartilage and bone, say nutritionists.

What You Can Do: While calcium is needed to fight osteoporosis, olive oil (which has a small amount of this mineral) can help supplement your intake of it when teamed with calcium-rich, bone-building foods.

8 **Defends Against HIV** In the early 1980s, HIV hit the world and caused a panic more than all of the above diseases combined

ever did. The question "What if it becomes a widespread epidemic?" haunted people around the world—of both genders. If you have human immunodeficiency virus (HIV), it can lead to acquired immune deficiency syndrome (AIDS), which can be spread to other people through the exchange of body fluids through sex, blood transfusions, and sharing of needles. There still is no cure.

How Olive Oil Works: While HIV—the cause of AIDS—has led to countless deaths globally, a new buzz is circulating. A compound called maslinic acid (a natural product derived from olive-pomace oil) may help to slow down the spread of HIV.

Researchers at the University of Granada believe that olive-pomace oil can slow down the spread of AIDS in the body by 80 percent. The product inhibits serine protease (an enzyme used by HIV to spread the infection throughout the body).

What You Can Do: Include olive oil in a well-balanced, nutrient-rich diet to keep your immune system in working order and fight off infections.

In the next chapter, I'll show you how the Mediterranean diet and its components, such as olive oil, come into play for good health—and why following this diet and lifestyle for life can be a good change to make today for tomorrow for you, your children, and their children to follow. It truly seems to be a key to good health. (Also, in Chapter 12, "Antiaging Wonder Food," I'll explain how some of these diseases can be controlled with olive oil and other preventive measures.)

THE GOLDEN SECRETS TO REMEMBER

OLIVE OIL KEEPS THE DOCTOR AWAY

Disease	How Olive Oil Works
√ Heart disease	Polyphenols in extra virgin olive oil help to lower the risk of heart disease of all kinds.
√ Cancer	Phenols in extra virgin olive oil act as disease-fighting antioxidants to hinder the cancer process; oleic acid may reduce the growth of tumors.
√ Arthritis	Omega-3s in extra virgin olive oil may play a role in reducing aches and pains because they may have an anti-inflammatory effect.
√ Diabetes	Olive oil may cut the amount of "bad" LDL cholesterol as well as triglycerides in the blood, which may lower the risk of developing type 2 diabetes.
√ Pain	Oleocanthal in olive oil can stop inflammation similar to the way painkillers do.
√ Impaired memory	Monounsaturated acids maintain cell structure and membranes in the brain.
√ Osteoporosis	Olive oil helps calcium absorption, which is needed to beat bone loss.
√ HIV	Maslinic acid (a natural product derived from olive-pomace oil) may help to slow down HIV.

The Keys to the Mediterranean Diet

*Cleopatra and Nefertiti knew the wonderful effects
of olive oil. Natural cosmetics are in. The Mediterranean lifestyle is in, and, thanks to cooking
shows on television, olive oil is in. It's that simple.*
—Margot Hellmiss[1]

When I was in my twenties, I had a boyfriend who was a full-blooded
Italian. One of the traits he possessed was that he loved to cook good,
hearty Mediterranean food. I was living on a shoestring in a downtown
Victorian studio in San Jose, California. It was charming but sparse.
After all, I was a starving student. But when he prepared dinners, I al-
ways felt like royalty.

One night in particular, my personal chef began the process of making a spaghetti sauce to die for. The ingredients, fresh tomatoes, garlic,
onions, and olive oil, reminds me of the noteworthy prison dinner
scene in the film *Goodfellas*. In other words, it doesn't matter where
you live but it matters how you put together a meal that sizzles. The
heart and soul of the Mediterranean diet and lifestyle, whether you are
from Italy or Greece, make cooking and eating a decadent pleasure.

I bet you think I'm going to discuss the popular Mediterranean diet
books. Not me. I've discovered in my research that for thousands of

years, olive oil—and other key factors—have played a major role on the Greek island of Crete, where Cretes and other Greeks live longer than other people in the world.

In fact, according to the World Health Organization, in 2004, the life span of men and women in Greece ranked second, with Italy third. Japan was number one, and the United States trailed behind.[2]

It turns out that the way I've been eating for decades (that is, fruits, vegetables, potatoes, nuts, seeds, bread and other cereals, and yogurt) is nothing new. However, using more "good" olive oil and less "bad" saturated fat is new to me, since I'm a boomer of the 1950s, when meat and potatoes were a constant on the average dinner table.

The fascinating thing is, while olive oil is a fat (120 calories per tablespoon), and other foods in the Mediterranean diet are high in fat, heart disease is lower and the longevity rate higher in European countries such as Greece and Italy than in America, where our fat intake is often lower. This is called the "French paradox," and it continues to work for people who follow the traditional Mediterranean diet. But for those who stick to the American diet and eat "bad" fats, unwanted body fat is the end result.

FIGHT FAT WITH FAT

When I was in my early forties, I discovered that while I looked skinny, I was fat. I recall that at this time, I was working out at the gym on a regular basis. While I was eating plenty of vegetables, fruits, and whole grains, I skipped the fish and "good" fats. A bodybuilder, Anna, noticed that my muscle mass wasn't in tip-top shape. Plus, the gym's nutritionist measured my body fat—not good.

So, I tweaked my diet big-time. I dumped the butter I was putting on baked potatoes. The blue cheese salad dressing got tossed into the trash, too. I began to eat tuna, salmon, and eggs, and I drizzled vinegar and olive oil on my salads and sandwiches. As I continued my new, improved Mediterranean-type diet and lifestyle, teamed with faster long-distance walking and more serious weight lifting, within weeks I noticed a difference in my muscle definition. Not only did I lose 5 pounds, but I built muscle and had a new, improved body, with sculpted arms and legs as well as normal blood pressure. I give credit to losing the "bad" fats and welcoming fish, eggs, fat, and a new exercise routine—all part of the Mediterranean diet.

10 KEYS TO THE MEDITERRANEAN DIET

These dietary tips, straight from Oldways Preservation & Exchange Trust, will help you to get on the right track to following a healthful, heart-healthy Mediterranean diet without feeling like you're on a diet.

TIP 1: Eat plenty of food from plant sources, including fruits and vegetables, potatoes, breads and grains, beans, nuts, and seeds.

TIP 2: Focus on a variety of minimally processed and, wherever possible, seasonally fresh and locally grown foods to get health-boosting and disease-fighting antioxidants.

TIP 3: Use olive oil as a primary fat, replacing other fats and oils (including butter and margarine).

TIP 4: Aim for a daily total fat amount ranging from about 25 to 35 percent of energy, with saturated fat composing no more than 7 to 8 percent of calories.

TIP 5: Consume low to moderate amounts of cheese and yogurt (low-fat and non-fat versions are best).

TIP 6: Eat low to moderate amounts of fish and poultry, and zero to four eggs per week (including those used in cooking and baking).

TIP 7: Enjoy fresh fruit as your daily dessert, and limit sweets with a sugar (often honey) or saturated fat to no more than a few times per week.

TIP 8: Consume red meat a few times per month. Lean cuts are preferable.

TIP 9: Get regular exercise, which will help you maintain a healthy weight, fitness, and well-being.

TIP 10: If you drink alcohol, opt for moderate consumption of wine, normally with meals. Limit intake to about one to two glasses per day for men and one glass per day for women. Note: Alcohol should be avoided during pregnancy and whenever it would put the individual at risk.

The Traditional Healthy Mediterranean Diet Pyramid

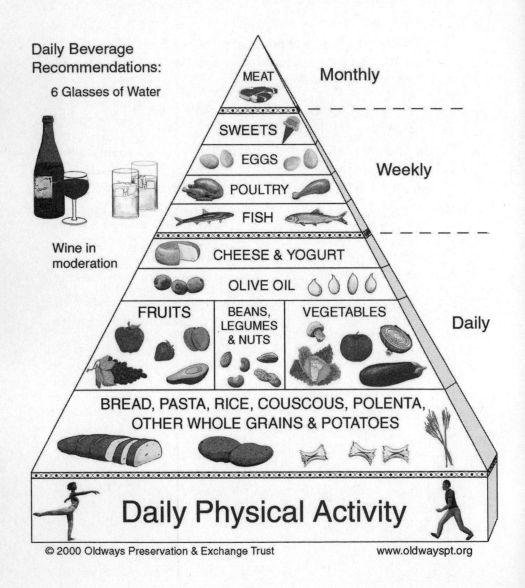

Daily Beverage Recommendations:

6 Glasses of Water

Wine in moderation

MEAT — Monthly

SWEETS

EGGS

POULTRY — Weekly

FISH

CHEESE & YOGURT

OLIVE OIL

FRUITS | BEANS, LEGUMES & NUTS | VEGETABLES — Daily

BREAD, PASTA, RICE, COUSCOUS, POLENTA, OTHER WHOLE GRAINS & POTATOES

Daily Physical Activity

© 2000 Oldways Preservation & Exchange Trust   www.oldwayspt.org

GOOD-FOR-YOU FOODS OF THE MEDITERRANEAN DIET

- *Bread, pasta, grains:* Bread, pasta, rice, couscous, polenta, potatoes
- *Fruits:* Olives, avocados, grapes
- *Vegetables:* Spinach, eggplant, tomatoes, broccoli, peppers, mushrooms, garlic, capers, beans, legumes, nuts, pine nuts, almonds, chickpeas, white beans, lentils, olive oil
- *Cheese and yogurt*
- *Fish:* Shellfish, sardines
- *Poultry:* Chicken
- *Eggs*
- *Sweets:* Pastries, ice cream, cookies
- *Meat:* Veal, lamb

In addition, daily physical activity is recommended. Getting physical can include doing chores, group activities, solo activities, fun stuff, and gym workouts. In other words, everyday lifestyle activities teamed with exercise is good for you head to toe, according to researchers and doctors.

Olive Oil on the Side

There are easy ways to fit an hour's worth of exercise (up to 500 calories burned) throughout your day by dividing it up into 10- or 15-minute segments. Just rev up your energy when doing everyday housework or chores—and don't forget the olive oil.

Chores	Calories Burned per 30 minutes	Olive Oil
Sitting (watching TV)	30	Read *The Healing Powers of Olive Oil* and learn new ways to maintain your weight

Chores	Calories Burned per 30 minutes	Olive Oil
Sleeping	30	Put olive oil on your feet
Washing the dog	97	Use a tablespoon of olive oil before shampooing
Raking leaves	98	Use olive oil on the rake to prevent rust
Painting the house	136	Use olive oil to remove paint from your skin
Chopping wood	150	Use olive oil–based soap afterward
Mowing the lawn	178	Use olive oil on the mower to prevent rust
Gardening	180	Spray indoor plants with olive oil and water
Scrubbing the floor	188	Use a solution of water and olive oil to clean the floor
Shoveling snow	195	Eat a pasta dish with olive oil for energy

According to the American Heart Association, "there's no one 'Mediterranean' diet. At least 16 countries border the Mediterranean Sea. Diets vary between these countries and also between regions within a county." However, the people of these various Mediterranean countries share these dietary components: high consumption of fruits, vegetables, bread and other cereals, potatoes, beans, nuts, and seeds; olive oil as an important monounsaturated fat source; dairy products, fish, and poultry consumed in low to moderate amounts and little red meat eaten; eggs consumed zero to four times a week; and wine consumed in low to moderate amounts.[3]

While the Mediterranean-style diets are similar to what the AHA recommends, they are not identical. In other words, the diets of the Mediterranean region do contain a high percentage of calories from fat. This is believed to be the cause of an increase of obesity in these countries.

The AHA points out that both heart disease and life span in the Mediterranean countries are lower than in the United States. They also note that "but this may not entirely be due to the diet. Lifestyle factors (such as more physical activity and extended social support systems) may also play a part." Before the AHA advises people to turn to the Mediterranean diet, more research is needed.

While I believe olive oil plays a big role in good health, I have also shown you that it's just part of the health package—it is not the only reason Europeans have lower rates of heart disease than Americans. Also, olive oil is ranked high as a superior healing oil, but take a look at Part 3, "Other Natural Oils," to see how olive oil's cousins—flavored oils (herbal, spice, vegetable, citrus, and other fruits) and other types of healing oils—can help you in other remarkable ways, too.

THE GOLDEN SECRETS TO REMEMBER

✓ Research shows that a low-fat diet does not lower health risks.
✓ The "French paradox," or eating a diet richer in fat combined with antioxidant-rich fruits and vegetables, may help lower your risk of developing cancer and heart disease.
✓ Research shows there is no reason to deprive yourself of "good" fatty foods such as fish and olive oil.

✓ The Mediterranean diet—food from plant sources—can help stave off heart disease.
✓ The Mediterranean diet includes using olive oil as a primary fat.
✓ Regular exercise and moderate consumption of wine (if you drink) are also included in the traditional healthy Mediterranean diet.

PART 3

OTHER NATURAL OILS

Flavored Olive Oils

The strands of spaghetti were vital, almost alive in
my mouth, and the olive oil was singing with flavor.
—Lucien Tendret[1]

Combine fresh herbs and spices with olive oil and what do you get? Healthful flavored or infused olive oils can offer an extra punch to your health and taste buds. Just ask Jonathan Sciabica, a member of the Sciabica family, which is well-known in the olive oil world for their products. He had this to say about their jalapeño olive oil: "This innovative combination of fresh jalapeños and Mission olives is a break from any conventional olive oil. Nick Jr. enjoys using this olive oil to fry his eggs in the morning. This won't really burn your tongue like a jalapeño might but you'll get a kick, and the flavor of the pepper comes through in the most amazing way."

Like healing olive oil, popular herbs and spices—such as jalapeño, oregano, and rosemary—boast health benefits, too. You can make your own flavored oils and reap a variety of therapeutic rewards from these herbs and spices mixed with extra virgin olive oil. Plus, it's most likely a rewarding experience to make your own flavored concoctions—sort of like growing your own vegetable garden.

Interestingly, "Olive oil which has had herbs or fruits infused in it cannot be called olive oil. According to International Olive Oil Council regulations it must be called 'fruit juice.' In reality, few producers comply with this and you will see labels such as 'lemon infused olive oil' or 'basil olive oil.' Because of their immense popularity, the California Olive Oil Council is trying to come up with a meaningful labeling standard for flavored oils," explains John Deane, M.D.

Meanwhile, I took Gemma Sciabica's advice and combined herbal, spice, and fruit "olive oils" in one chapter. At first, I was going to discuss herbal oils and fruit-flavored oils in separate chapters. So, read on—and discover some of the delicious concoctions you can add to your diet.

HEALING HERBAL AND SPICE OILS

Here, take a look at some of the favorite and cutting-edge herbs and spices that are infused in olive oil, as well as some information and news about their healing powers.

CHICORY (*Cichorium intybus*): The Eygptians and Greeks drank roasted chicory root to relieve stomach, liver, and kidney complaints. A tonic made from chicory root is believed to increase the flow of bile, which is good for staying regular.

GARLIC (*Allium sativum*): It's an ancient healing food. During biblical times, garlic was praised for its versatile uses, including as a diuretic, a sedative, an anti-inflammatory, and a cure for internal parasites, and in poultices.

JAPALEÑO (*Capsicum annuum*): It's capsaicin, the hot stuff, that may help slow down cancer cell growth, clear sinus congestion, soothe a migraine, act as an anti-inflammatory, and make aches and pains go away. Hot peppers also have antioxidants A, C, and E.

OREGANO (*Oregano vulgare*): Oregano oil is both antiseptic and anti-inflammatory. Not only does it kill bacteria, viruses, fungi, and other germs, but it also fights infection, from colds to the flu.

PARSLEY (*Petroselinum crispum*): Parsley can be traced back to Greek mythology. Legend has it that it was a bad omen for a soldier to see it before going to battle. But things have changed. This cleansing herb is packed with disease-fighting antioxidant vitamins A, C, and E.

Also, it boasts plenty of iron. Parsley gets its good reputation, however, for its diuretic action. Plus, it's believed to ease PMS symptoms, including cramps, hormonal mood swings, and bloating.

ROSEMARY (*Rosmarinus officinalis*): Rosemary is believed to cure headaches, hemorrhoids, depression, and other ailments that take a toll on your total health and well-being. This ancient therapeutic herb contains calcium, magnesium, sodium, and potassium, all of which help balance fluids surrounding the nerves and heart tissues. In fact, rosemary may help to lower blood pressure. The rosemary leaf may also have other positive health effects.

SAGE (*Salvia officinalis*): This camphor-flavored "fountain of youth" grows wild in the Mediterranean. Its Latin name means "to heal or save." Legend has it that sage will add years to a person's life if used regularly. Herbalists claim sage is a natural astringent and antiseptic. It's recommended for gingivitis and sore throats. Note, however, that women should not take it.

THYME (*Thymus vulgaris*): Thyme is a delicate herb that is a natural source of iron, magnesium, silicon, sodium, and thiamine. Its power is as an antiseptic and a general healing tonic. It can also subdue coughing and relieve intestinal ailments.

Make Your Own Flavored Olive Oils

You can purchase ready-made infused olive oils or make your own flavored oils by blending your favorite herbs and spices. The safest way is to use dried herbs. Sure, you can use fresh ingredients (and actually, I would prefer to do just that), but caution is advised. Why? Simply put, it's risky business to put anything in the oil that contains water. That means, be on alert when teaming olive oil with garlic, lemon peel, fresh peppers, fresh herbs, or spices. The fact is, the oil won't support bacterial growth, but the water-containing herbs will. Worse, botulism bacteria can grow in this type of environment. (Yes, botulism can make you very ill.) But note, there are several ways to have your homemade flavored oils and survive, too. Here, take a glance at four tips that can help you do it yourself:

- Mix all the ingredients. Then, put the prepared oil in the fridge and use it within one week. Go ahead—add whole cloves of garlic, lemon peel, fresh or dried peppers, ginger, rosemary sprigs, or whatever strikes your fancy.
- Preserve the added ingredients. Maybe you have seen garlic or herbs mixed with olive oil. The way it is done commercially is to first preserve the water-containing garlic or herb in a strong brine or vinegar solution, then put it in the olive oil. The vinegar solutions used commercially are up to four times stronger than the vinegars you find in the supermarket. You can find them at commercial food supply outlets. Many of the herb mixes have both salt and vinegar, both of which prevent bacterial growth.
- Dry the herbs to remove all the water, leaving the essential oils. This can be done using a food dehydrator or just by leaving them in the sun. Then, add the spices and herbs to the olive oil.
- Press the olives with the spices. Putting lemon, garlic, and other ingredients in the olive press with the olives is the safest way to flavor olive oil. *Note:* The glitch is that you have to have your own olive press or go to a commercial press. The oils from the added ingredients mix with the olive oil, and the watery parts of the spices are removed along with the olive water. You can mix a small amount of oil with the fresh ingredients, let the flavors mingle, and then decant the oil, leaving the herbs and any water behind. Mix this flavored oil with a larger amount of oil. You can also add essential spice oils to the olive oil to achieve the same effect.

(*Source:* John Deane, M.D.)

Warning: It is difficult to determine the exact shelf life of homemade flavored olive oils. American Dietetic Association (ADA) nutritionists question their safety, since we do not know if we can prevent food-borne illnesses. So caution is advised.

HEALING CITRUS OILS

Citrus olive oils—lemon, lime, orange, and tangerine—are new and exciting to me. Personally, I have already tried a commercial brand of lemon olive oil. One night, I tossed some in a pasta dish. While it wasn't homemade, it did add zest to my pasta plate. Still, there is a wide world of citrus olive oils . . .

I do know that lemon—a fresh, light, and cool scent—was used in ancient times to perfume clothes and repel insects. Europeans used lemons to fight infectious illnesses such as malaria, and English sailors turned to lemons as a scurvy remedy. You can use lemon for its light and zingy benefits. If you're feeling down and blue, it can pick up your spirits. This oil is used in beauty products, soaps, and household cleansers.

One man in particular really knows his flavored oils, and it shows in his book *Michael Chiarello's Flavored Oils and Vinegars* (Chronicle Books, 2006). He writes, "Some lemon oils made in Tuscany are extraordinary. Whole lemons are ground along with the olives into a paste and then pressed, extracting the lemon flavor with the oil. In this process, the lemon and olive flavors become joined in a way impossible to duplicate in the home kitchen. These oils also tend to be fabulously expensive. Home-made oils emphasize the fresh, juicy character of citrus and are a particular delight for summer cooking."[2]

Here, take a look at an easy-to-do lemon olive oil recipe that spells "fresh" from the get-go.

Lemon Olive Oil

1 lemon
2 cups Marsala Olive Fruit Oil

Peel lemon with vegetable peeler. Place peel and olive oil in glass container and cover. Bring to room temperature before serving. Keep refrigerated for several days. Bring to room temperature before serving.

(*Source: Cooking with California Olive Oil: Treasured Family Recipes* by Gemma Sanita Sciabica)

Chiarello explains in his book that the flavors of citrus oils "are essentially interchangeable." I suppose that is true unless you happen to love lemon and lime as I do. But in a pinch, the flavored olive oil is all right. "If I run out of orange," he says, "I just fill out the amount in the recipe with lemon. When using citrus oil, you are adding the flavor but not the acid."[3]

I'm not surprised that Chiarello adds that citrus oils are superb when paired with salads—and you don't need vinegar. Also, he adds that citrus-flavored olive oils are different from the concentrated citrus essence oils on the market and that you can't use them in the same ways, such as in baking, to flavor cakes and cookies. (I almost used lemon olive oil in baking a batch of brownies, but ended up purchasing extra virgin olive oil. I'm glad I did.)

Now that we've put some favorite flavored oils on the table (in Chapter 18, "The Joy of Cooking with Olive Oil," discover which foods go best with flavored olive oils), let's talk about other healing oils that are used inside and outside the body.

THE GOLDEN SECRETS TO REMEMBER

✓ Chicory	Relieves stomach, liver, kidney ailments
✓ Garlic	An anti-inflammatory, a diuretic, a sedative
✓ Jalapeño	Slows cancer growth, clears sinuses, soothes aches
✓ Oregano	Antiseptic and anti-inflammatory, relieves muscle soreness
✓ Parsley	Cleanser, diuretic
✓ Rosemary	Heart-healthy, cancer-fighting
✓ Sage	Astringent, antiseptic, soothes sore throats
✓ Thyme	Antiseptic, helps anemia, suppresses coughs, relieves stomach upsets

8

More Healing Oils

We know consumers recognize the various types of dietary fats but have a hard time determining what types to increase or decrease in their diet. This provides an opportunity to encourage consumers to choose foods rich in healthful fats such as plant-based oils.

—Susan T. Borra[1]

In my college days—the first time around, in junior college—I recall taking a nutrition class. I was fascinated with calories and staying fit (it was in the 1970s, and staying clear of fat and looking skinny like fashion models in *Cosmopolitan* and *Vogue* magazines was "in"). But, I flunked the lesson on fats. I remember it was confusing—fats such as saturated, polyunsaturated, and monounsaturated. At the time, to me, it was boring. It was a foreign language.

TALKING "GOOD" FATS IS IN STYLE

These days, people around the world are talking about "good" fat. Not only is olive oil hot stuff, but other oils are now also the talk of the town. Why? Food chains from Starbucks to Kentucky Fried Chicken (KFC) are jumping on the "good"-fats bandwagon and deleting trans fats—and choosing other types of oils for their fried and baked foods.

KFC, for one, is turning to a new soybean oil—a neutral-tasting, all-purpose, organic oil. Soybean oil contains both omega-3 and omega-6 fats as well as good-for-you monounsaturated fat and saturated fat. To reach zero trans fat, Starbucks is replacing butter with a trans-fat-free margarine and a butter–trans-fat-free margarine blend. "There is, however, the possibility that certain items may have trans-fat-free vegetable oils (such as soy or canola oil) but this is not broadly used in our fresh baked products," said company spokesperson Alan Hilowitz.

So, now that popular food chains are getting fat-savvy, read on to get a handle on some of the cooking oils. (See Chapter 11, "The Olive Oil Diet," to learn more about how unhealthy trans fats can not only be harmful for heart health, but can pack on the pounds, too.)

ALL FATS ARE NOT CREATED EQUAL

Type of Fat	Oils	Effects on Your Body
Saturated	Coconut oil, palm kernel oil	Raises both LDL and HDL cholesterol
Polyunsaturated	Vegetable oils: corn, sesame, soybean	Reduces both HDL and LDL cholesterol; too much may raise cancer risk
Monounsaturated	Canola oil, olive oil, peanut oil	Lowers LDL, HDL stays the same or may be raised depending upon the individual
Trans fatty acid	Margarines, vegetable shortenings	Raises LDL, lowers HDL

COMMON COOKING OILS

Canola Oil

Oil Roots: Canola, also called rapeseed, was made back in the 1970s from mustard rape, which has been used for more than three thousand years. The term "canola" was coined by the Canadian government for "canada oil."

Healing Powers: Canola oil has the lowest level of artery-clogging saturated fat and is rich in monounsaturated fats, the good stuff that helps keep your blood cholesterol in check. As for olive oil, 1 tablespoon contains about 120 calories and 14 grams of total fat. However, canola oil is lower in saturated fat: it contains 1 gram versus 2 grams in olive oil. Still, the oil gets a stamp of approval with an FDA heart health claim.

Best Uses: Canola oil is a good cooking oil, such as for stir-fries and sautéing. It doesn't cost as much as extra virgin olive oil. High monosaturated oils like canola are good all-purpose oils, since they can take higher heat than polyunsaturated oils such as safflower, sunflower, and soybean.

Chefs will tell you that extra virgin olive oil and canola oil pair up well in the kitchen. Since the strong flavor in extra virgin olive oil dissipates when sustained heat is used, it is advised to use this pricey oil for salad dressings and sautés and as a tasty condiment, while reserving neutral-flavored canola oil for use with up to medium high heat (375°F).

Lorenzo's Oil (Olive and Rapeseed Oil)

Remember the 1992 film *Lorenzo's Oil*? The story is about an uncommon debilitating disorder called adrenoleukodystrophy (ALD), which, in nearly half of cases, destroys the nerves in the brain. Young boys who are affected, such as Lorenzo Odone, usually become disabled (it can look like multiple sclerosis) and often die sooner than later.

One remedy is Lorenzo's oil, which is made from olive and rapeseed oils, teamed with a low-fat diet. While the oil has not been proven to be a wonder drug, Lorenzo Odone celebrated his twenty-eighth birthday in 2006. According to the www.washingtonpost.com, on January 28, 2007, Lorenzo was still alive at 28. I don't know if he is alive today or will be in 2008.

Interestingly, rapeseed oil, a monounsaturated fat, is high in both omega-3 and omega-6 fats. Still, the "healing" oil has a bad reputation on some Internet sites that have linked the oil to causing health problems, due to its component of erucic acid. Some people are also concerned about canola oil, which has a very low level of erucic acid.

Coconut Oil

Oil Roots: It has been touted as a "healthy" oil in tropical regions as well as sold in the South Seas and South Asian markets as far back as the mid-nineteenth century.

Healing Powers: Coconut oil has a variety of uses. It has been known to have antiviral and antimicrobial benefits due to its lauric acid content. Also, its fatty components—caprylic and lauric acids—may support immune function. It has been used for candida and yeast infections.

Best Uses: Coconut oil is used for beauty care. It may also help moisturize skin and hair. Using coconut oil as an alternative to butter or unhealthy trans fats, in conjunction with a healthy diet plan and regular exercise, may help you lose weight, but it is not a magic bullet, according to Spectrum Naturals. And note, while coconut oil can be used as an alternative to butter, margarine, and shortening in cooking and baking using up to medium heat, 1 tablespoon contains 12 grams of saturated fat so you will want to limit your consumption of it.

Evening Primrose Oil

Oil Roots: The evening primrose (*Oenothera biennis*)—a plant with bright yellow flowers—is found in dry meadows from the Atlantic to the Rocky Mountains. It blooms only in the evening—hence the name "evening primrose"—then dies, leaving seed pods, which can be used for their oil.

Healing Powers: Evening primrose oil contains gamma-linolenic acid (GLA), an essential fatty acid. Some medical experts believe GLA is the most important essential oil for treating PMS and menopausal symptoms.

Research suggests that women with PMS or menopausal woes have low levels of GLA. It's been theorized that such a deficiency might cause a prostaglandin deficiency and trigger a sensitivity to prolactin, the pituitary hormone. GLA supplementation may relieve the prostaglandin deficiency.

Not only is prolactin involved in the menstrual cycle and the ending of it, so are the hormones progesterone and estrogen, which can affect water retention, breast swelling, irritability, and breast tenderness. The GLA from evening primrose oil may help to balance these fluctuating hormone levels.

Best Uses: Many women take evening primrose oil capsules fourteen days before their period to relieve PMS symptoms. Evening primrose oil is found in health food stores.

Fish Oil

Oil Roots: Eskimos in Alaska and Greenland eat cold water fatty fish as a staple in their diet. This has resulted in their having fewer problems with cancer and heart disease, which affect people who use unhealthy fats.

Healing Powers: Fish oil is rich in the omega-3 fatty acids EPA and DHA. Fish oil can be helpful for arthritis because the omega-3 oils are important in the lubrication of the joints. They also reduce pro-inflammatory chemicals called prostaglandins. Some holistic doctors believe that a diet high in the essential fatty acids is brain food. EFAs can help the cell membranes work in the brain.

The omega-3s are diabetes fighters because they can help control the blood sugar and help prevent damage to all tissues. Also, the omega-3s are essential fatty acids that have protective effects on heart disease. And, not surprisingly, Dr. Barry Sears' *Omega Rx Zone: The Miracle of the New High Dose Fish Oil* (Regan Books, 2002) touts fish oil for better health.

Best Uses: Fish oil capsules are taken as a supplement and are helpful for people who do not get an adequate amount of the omega-3 fatty acids EPA and DHA. But note, do not take high doses of fish capsules if you are taking NSAIDs (nonsteroidal anti-inflammatory drugs). They may increase gastrointestinal ulcers and bleeding.

Supplement Facts Fish Oil Serving Size 2 Softgels	
Amount per serving	%Daily Value
Calories 20	
Calories from fat 20	
Total fat 2 g	3%
Saturated fat 0.5 g	3%
Trans fat 0 g	
Polyunsaturated fat 1 g	
Monounsaturated fat 1g	
Cholesterol 12 mg	4%
Vitamin A 200 IU	4%
Omega-3 800 mg	
EPA (eicosapentaenoic acid) 360 mg	277%
DHA (docosahexaenoic acid) 240 mg	185%
Omega-6 50 mg	
Omega-9 (oleic acid OA) 185 mg	

*Percent Daily Values (DV) are based on a 2,000 calorie diet.
Source: Spectrum Naturals.

Flaxseed Oil

Oil Roots: Flaxseed was discovered as a food by the Greeks and the Romans. This plant with turquoise blue blossoms is hailed because of the oil that comes from its seeds and the many health virtues that oil provides.

Healing Powers: Flaxseed oil is Mother Nature's best source of alpha-linolenic acid, an omega-3 essential fatty acid—the same healthful fatty acid in fish oil that boosts heart health, reduces inflammation, and enhances cell function in your body. Medical experts also believe it can be a woman's best friend. Why? It has been known to aid in PMS and menopausal woes. It also lowers cholesterol and blood pressure, and may help lower the risk of developing heart attack and stroke.[2]

Best Uses: Flavorful flax oil can be a healthful replacement for butter. But note, it is not good for cooking because high heat will destroy the good-for-you nutrients of the oil. Go ahead and use this oil as a flavoring for potatoes, vegetables, and popcorn. Also, nutritionists recommend adding flax oil to smoothies, yogurt, and salad dressing.

Supplement Facts Flaxseed Oil, Organic Serving Size 1 Tablespoon (14 g)	
Amount per serving	%Daily Value
Calories 130	
Calories from fat 130	
Total fat 14 g	22%
Saturated fat 1.5 g	6%
Trans fat 0 g	
Polyunsaturated fat 10 g	
Monounsaturated fat 3 g	
Omega-3 (alpha-linolenic acid ALA) 8 g	615%
Omega-6 (linoleic acid LA) 2 g	
Omega-9 (oleic acid OA) 3 g	
*Percent Daily Values (DV) are based on a 2,000 calorie diet. *Source:* Spectrum Naturals.	

Grapeseed Oil

Oil Roots: Grapeseed oil (also called grape oil) has been used for thousands of years by people in European countries. These days, grapeseed is produced in Italy, France, and Spain. Its versatile appeal has made it a common oil for cooking and baking, to make flavored oils, and massage oils, and in hair products, lip balm, hand creams, and sunburn repair lotions.

Healing Powers: It's rich in antioxidants, which can help fight diseases such as cancer and heart disease. In fact, it may help to lower cholesterol levels, according to studies conducted by cardiologists.

Best Uses: Grapeseed oil can be used for sautéing, medium-high-heat frying, and baking. [and oil infusing (i.e. flavored oils).] Grapeseed oil is excellent for cooking, since it can be brought to a higher heat and has a milder taste than extra virgin olive oil.

Nutrition Facts Grapeseed Oil, Refined
Serving Size 1 tablespoon (14 g)
Amount per serving
Calories 120
Calories from fat 120
Total fat 14 g
Trans fat 0 g
Cholesterol 0 mg
Polyunsaturated fat 10 g
Monounsaturated fat 3 g
Sodium 0 mg
Potassium 0 mg
Total Carbohydrate 0 g
Source: Adapted from Spectrum Naturals.

OILS AT A GLANCE

Medical doctors, nutritionists, and chefs will tell you that olive oil is not the only healing oil, since the following oils have great benefits, too.

Oil	What It Does
Canola oil	A popular oil, like olive oil, that is rich in monounsaturated fat. It contains heart-healthy omega-3s.
Coconut oil	An oil that is healthful for your outer body beauty, from hair to skin, because of its rich moisturizing benefits.

Oil	What It Does
Evening primrose oil	An oil that is beneficial for fighting irritability, mood changes, anxiety, fluid retention, and even sleep disorders.
Fish oil	An oil rich in fatty acids, omega-3s, and omega-6s that can support the entire body's system. Omega-3s help control blood sugar, help prevent damage to all tissues, and control plaque blockage to prevent stroke.
Flaxseed oil	A high-lignan oil that relieves depression, fatigue, and allergies. Lignans are estrogen-like substances that have balancing effects on serotonin and other mood regulators.
Grapeseed oil	An antioxidant-rich oil that may help prevent diseases such as cancer and high cholesterol.

MORE COOKING OILS FYI

There are many other cooking oils that you should be familiar with so you can have a variety to use for fun and good health. Here, take a look at other heart-healthy oils:

- *Almond oil, refined:* A high-heat cooking oil rich in heart-healthy monounsaturated fats.
- *Apricot oil, refined:* A French oil for high-heat sautés.
- *Avocado oil, refined:* A good oil for heat; a monounsaturated fat.
- *Corn oil, unrefined:* An oil with a rich flavor, good for any dish, from pancakes to pasta.
- *Peanut oil, unrefined:* An oil that adds depth and intensity to sautés and stir-fries.
- *Safflower oil, refined, organic:* A light, neutral-flavored oil that's a natural in the kitchen.
- *High-heat safflower oil, organic, refined:* An oil that's higher in monounsaturated fat and lower in both saturated and polyunsaturated fats than regular sunflower oil, which means it's good for your heart and for high-heat cooking.

- *Sesame oil, unrefined, organic:* An oil that makes your stir-fries come alive—use an unrefined version for especially true flavor.
- *Soy oil, refined, organic:* A neutral-tasting, all-purpose, organic oil.
- *Walnut oil, refined:* A good way to introduce omega-3s into your kitchen. Try it drizzled over endive scattered with blue cheese and toasted nuts.

Source: Spectrum Naturals.

Note: Check with your doctor before using any of these oils in case there's a medical reason they're not right for you.

Speaking of healing oils, in Part 4, "Youth in a Bottle," you'll learn how teaming vinegars (especially apple cider vinegar and red wine vinegar) with olive oil is another Mediterranean secret to losing body fat, maintaining your weight, and stalling age-related diseases such as heart disease.

THE GOLDEN SECRETS TO REMEMBER

- ✓ Saturated oils—such as coconut oil and palm kernel oil—aren't heart-healthy, so be sure to use them in moderation.
- ✓ Polyunsaturated oils—vegetable oils such as corn and sesame—reduce "bad" cholesterol, but using too much can up your risk for developing cancer.
- ✓ Monounsaturated oils—canola oil and olive oil—are the healthiest fats.
- ✓ Trans fatty acids—margarines and vegetable shortenings—are unhealthy, artery-clogging fats that can cause heart disease and weight gain.
- ✓ Canola oil contains heart-healthy omega-3s and is a good fat choice.
- ✓ Evening primrose oil and flaxseed oil are good oils for women because they can help in coping with hormonal woes such as PMS and menopausal symptoms.
- ✓ Fish oil—rich in both omega-3s and omega-6s—can help prevent heart disease, diabetes, and other health problems.

✓ Grapeseed oil, high in disease-fighting antioxidants, can stave off heart disease and cancer.

✓ There is a wide variety of cooking oils that include fruits, nuts, and soy.

✓ Some nut oils, such as almond oil and walnut oil, are heart-healthy.

PART 4

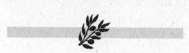

YOUTH IN A BOTTLE

Combining Olive Oil and Vinegar

*If you pour oil and vinegar into the same vessel,
you would call them not friends but opponents.*
—Aeschylus[1]

Since biblical times, oil, like vinegar, which was known as "the poor man's wine," has played a role in the lives of both the rich, such as royalty, and the poor. In the popular legend of the Four Thieves, the robbers are believed to have used powerful vinegar and herbs to beat getting the deadly plague. But, some olive oil experts believe the savvy foursome used a healing-oil formula. Perhaps they used both oil and vinegar, which together have antiseptic and immunity-boosting properties.

OIL AND VINEGAR

A number of historical reports show that the ancient Babylonians favored oil-and-vinegar dressings. The ancient Egyptians left written accounts of various oil-and-vinegar dressings that included imported herbs and spices.[2]

In the twentieth century, people in the United States were able to purchase prepared dressings that included olive oil and vinegar along with spices and other ingredients. Some of the popular brands of salad dressings we use today go back as far as the early part of that century.

Today, in the twenty-first century, as you know, there are countless olive oils and vinegars on the market. Apple cider and red wine and balsamic vinegars and rice, fruit, and specialty vinegars are all used worldwide. But the fact remains, it's red wine vinegar and apple cider vinegar that seem to get the most credit, and for good reason.

Here, take a look at the two most popular vinegars. Not only were apple cider vinegar and red wine vinegar praised centuries ago, they still deserve praise today. There are many reasons why.

APPLE CIDER VINEGAR AND OLIVE OIL

Researchers are discovering that baby boomers are targets for metabolic syndrome, a cluster of conditions that increase the risk of stroke, diabetes, and heart attack.

Apple cider vinegar may be the perfect and practical modern miracle for baby boomers and seniors (and the younger generations). Metabolic syndrome can be hindered through the use of the simple apple cider vinegar found in your kitchen cupboard or refrigerator.

How? How can this vinegar fight metabolic syndrome? For starters, nutritionists say apple cider vinegar can help you to lose body fat, a culprit that can lead to cholesterol and triglyceride (blood fats) problems, high blood sugar, high blood pressure—all signs of metabolic syndrome.

So, how can apple cider vinegar help you burn fat instead of store it? Ann Louise Gittleman, Ph.D., C.N.S., gave me the plain and simple answer. "Apple cider is a notable fat burner because of its ability to keep sodium and potassium levels balanced. As a potassium-rich food, a couple of ounces of apple cider vinegar a day will put the lid on your appetite because you will be far less hungry and far less bloated."

Apple cider vinegar can help you lose inches faster than pounds, too. "Many individuals boast they shed inches more quickly than they pare pounds. This is again due to the high potassium levels which help to flush out water-logged tissues, created by excessive amounts of water-retaining sodium," adds Gittleman.

Also, organic apple cider vinegar made from fresh apples can contain a healthy dose of pectin. Soluble fiber may help lower "bad" cholesterol by binding with it. Your body then eliminates the fiber, say nutritionists. As a result, you may be able to reduce your risk of heart attack and stroke.

Apple Cider Vinegar, a Dieter's Best Friend

Three-and-one-half ounces of apple cider vinegar contains:

95 percent water
14 calories
0 grams protein
0 grams dietary fiber
0 grams fat
5 grams carbohydrates
6 milligrams calcium
9 milligrams phosphorus
0.6 milligram iron
1 milligram sodium
100 milligrams potassium
22 milligrams magnesium
0.04 milligram copper

Source: The Healing Powers of Vinegar.

In addition to adding vinegar to your diet, include olive oil, too. Here, take a look at some vinegar-and-oil weight loss tips:

1. Switch to a salad dressing of vinegar and extra virgin olive oil. One of the biggest sources of fat and calories in the average woman's diet is salad dressing. When you toss a salad of mixed greens, substitute 1 tablespoon each of extra virgin olive oil and vinegar.

2. You lose inches faster when you trim your sandwich, even just a little. Build a more slimming sandwich by substituting poultry for the meat and the cheese; adding plenty of fresh tomatoes, dark green lettuce, and onions; and replacing the mayonnaise with a splash of olive oil and vinegar.

3. Lose the butter and margarine. Giving up these two fats and replacing them with olive oil will make a big difference, not only in your weight loss, but in your heart health, too.

4. Instead of sautéing your vegetables in butter, try using an olive oil spray and a splash of vinegar to avoid adding unhealthy saturated fat to your diet.

5. Eating a Mediterranean-style diet—vegetables, fruits, grains, low-fat dairy, fish, and olive oil—can help you shed unwanted weight, but so can getting regular physical activity.

APPLE CIDER VINEGAR FIGHTS METABOLIC SYNDROME

Disease	How ACV Works
Diabetes	ACV in the diet may help to slow the rise of blood sugar after a high-carbohydrate meal.
Overweight	The fiber in ACV provides bulk and curbs appetite, keeps your sodium–potassium ratio in balance so you're less hungry, and decreases bloating and water retention.
High blood pressure	The potassium in ACV helps reduce hypertension, especially if you team it with potassium-rich fruits and vegetables.
High cholesterol	The insoluble fiber in ACV reduces cholesterol by binding with it. The fiber is then eliminated by the body.

RED WINE VINEGAR AND OLIVE OIL

According to researchers at Harvard University and the National Institute of Aging, resveratrol, an antioxidant found in red wine, inhibited the bad effects of a high-calorie diet in mice and added years to their life span. If people add red wine vinegar (which may contain heart-healthy resveratrol) along with resveratrol-rich foods such as peanuts, blueberries, cranberries, and plums—and olive oil—to their diets, can they stall Father Time?

Yes, it is possible. While apple cider vinegar and olive oil can fight body fat and heart disease, it's the Mediterranean-type red wine and balsamic vinegars teamed with a Mediterranean diet including olive oil that may also fight obesity, which is often linked to heart disease.

Red wine and balsamic vinegars are both derived from grapes. And like red wine, they contain disease-fighting antioxidants such as quercetin and (most likely) resveratrol, especially in the premium, organic brands. While studies have shown that drinking a glass of red wine daily can cut your heart disease risk, consuming these vinegars teamed with olive oil can give you all the same health benefits but without the alcohol. More research is needed to prove that red wine vinegar contains resveratrol. Meanwhile, using it with olive oil on foods that definitely contain resveratrol is a key to fighting metabolic syndrome and stalling age-related diseases.

RED WINE VINEGAR FIGHTS METABOLIC SYNDROME

Disease	How RWV Works
Diabetes	The quercetin in RWV slows the release of insulin.
Heart attack, stroke	The polyphenols in RWV slow down blood clotting by their antioxidant action; the resveratrol (if contained) prevents blood-platelet aggregation and increases HDL cholesterol levels; the tannins reduce platelet aggregation and increase HDL cholesterol levels.
Heart disease	The proanthocyanidins in RWV block the formation of cholesterol deposits on artery walls.
High cholesterol	The catechin in RWV blocks "bad" LDL cholesterol from entering the artery walls, inhibits blood clots from forming, relaxes blood vessels, and inhibits the development of tumors; the flavonoids may help reduce cholesterol levels and prevent the oxidation of LDL cholesterol.

A WEIGHT LOSS SUCCESS STORY

Meet Terry Flores, an Ohio-based, 42-year-old, busy married mom of three boys. One month, I called her and asked her if she wanted to follow my vinegar-based diet plan based on the Mediterranean diet lifestyle. She said that at 5 feet 5 inches and 197 pounds, she was willing to do it.

For two months, she drank a tablespoon of apple cider vinegar in an 8-ounce glass of water three to four times a day. "I also alternated adding red wine vinegar and apple cider vinegar to my meals and salads for flavor. When I cooked my meals with vegetables, fish, and chicken, I always used olive oil. The vegetable oil made it taste heavy, so I only use olive oil now."

While Terry did see almost immediate results, a few times she hit a diet plateau. Therefore, she turned to the Bloat-Busting Meal Plan about every other week. She blames her setbacks on the stress levels in her life, but vows her body responds to the jump-start two-day diet plan.

In two months, Terry lost 17 pounds and four dress sizes. Now at size 12/14, she is confident that she will be wearing a size 10 sooner than later. She says, "My husband and boys keep telling me how great I look. I even like what I see in the mirror again. I know I can do this. After seven years of trying to lose and not being able to, I have hope again."

Terry's Favorite Two-Day "Gut-Busting" Diet

This slimming, healthy meal plan—designed by New Jersey–based nutritionist Toni Gerbino—can help you to lose inches and pare pounds. Also, if you reach that dieter's plateau where the scale numbers won't budge, this is a great way to get back on track.

Breakfast:
  Fresh berries (no limit)

Lunch:
  4 ounces fresh white meat turkey
  Greens with dressing made of fresh parsley, 1 tablespoon each virgin olive oil and apple cider vinegar, and spices to taste
  1 cup fresh berries

Dinner:

   6 to 8 ounces fresh flounder, sole, or salmon
   Asparagus with lemon, apple cider vinegar, and parsley
   1 cup fresh berries

Drink a minimum of six 8-ounce glasses of water with fresh lemon throughout the day.
   Note: Check with your doctor before starting this or any diet.

Red Wine Vinegar Marinade for Meat and Poultry

❖ ❖ ❖

⅓ cup Spectrum Naturals Organic Red Wine Vinegar
3 cloves garlic, finely minced
1 teaspoon each fresh thyme leaves, fresh rosemary leaves, and fresh parsley leaves

⅓ cup dry red wine (optional)
½ cup Spectrum Naturals Organic Extra Virgin Olive Oil
1 teaspoon salt
1 teaspoon freshly ground black pepper

Combine all the ingredients. Pour over meat or poultry, and let marinate for 4 to 8 hours. Makes 1 cup.

Terry's Diet-Plateau Blasters

While Terry did lose weight, she also hit several diet plateaus. Upon her request, I provided her with these bonus weight-loss tips to help her continue to lose unwanted pounds. These 15 tips are based on the Mediterranean diet and lifestyle.

1. Do eat breakfast every day. It jump-starts your metabolism, provides energy, and staves off hunger pangs to help you stay clear of overeating.

2. Do not eat after 7 P.M. If you must eat something, try a piece of fresh fruit and a cup of herbal tea.

3. Forgo foods with trans fats or partially hydrogenated oils (for ex-

ample, packaged foods such as muffins, cakes, and cookies), which can lead to weight gain.

4. Instead, eat fresh foods (whole grains, fruits, vegetables, fish, legumes, unsalted nuts, and olive oil).

5. Practice portion control. Forget second helpings or eating 6 ounces of fish instead of 3 ounces. Again, read labels. A cup of yogurt is one serving. An orange or apple should be small or medium, not a giant whopper.

6. When you exercise, up your time by 15 minutes, or increase the intensity if you are doing calorie-burning aerobics.

7. Try working out with weights, which can help boost your metabolism for hours after you are done.

8. On a non-stressful day (or on a stressful one), try a juice-and-vegetable detox diet. It will cleanse your system and allow you more energy and less weight the next day.

9. If you eat white bread, white pasta, or white rice, make the switch to whole wheat, which has more filling fiber.

10. Don't get on the scale every day. Building muscle and losing inches is more important than losing pounds. Sooner than later, your body will rebuild itself if you remain true to a healthful diet and exercise.

11. Wear loose-fitting clothing, which will allow you to be more active and comfortable.

12. That spaghetti sauce? It's too high in sodium, which can make you retain water. Dump it, and substitute tomato paste.

13. Speaking of sodium, potassium-rich fruits and vegetables can help you lose water weight. Make sure you get five to nine servings daily, and drizzle them with olive oil.

14. Watch your sodium intake. Lose the canned foods, lunch meats, cheese, all of which contain sodium, which also can raise your blood pressure.

15. Make sure you take a vitamin-mineral supplement daily to ensure you get the essential vitamins and minerals.

Bonus tip: Drink six to eight 8-ounce glasses of spring water each day. They will help keep you hydrated, energized, and satisfied.

THE GOLDEN SECRETS TO REMEMBER

✓ Oil and vinegar were paired back in ancient history.
✓ In the twentieth century, store-bought dressings teamed oil and vinegar.
✓ Today, in the twenty-first century, health-conscious consumers purchase oil and vinegar separately and marry the foods to keep the result low in sodium, low in calories, and better in quality.
✓ Apple cider vinegar and olive oil can help fight metabolic syndrome, a problem in boomers and seniors that can lead to heart attack, stroke, diabetes, and obesity.
✓ Red wine vinegar and olive oil—with its polyphenol content— can help cut your risk of developing heart disease and obesity.
✓ You can use olive oil to help you jump-start a diet or break a plateau.

The Elixir to Heart Health

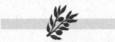

*One tablespoon of olive oil has the power to wipe
out the cholesterol raising effects of two eggs.*
—Jean Carper[1]

In addition to keeping you lean and fit, eating heart-healthy foods can also help to cut your risk of developing heart disease. So can eating "good" fats—essential fatty acids. That's what medical doctors will tell you—years ago, today, and most likely in years to come.

In my mid-forties, my blood pressure and cholesterol weren't a big concern. But now, like countless baby boomers and seniors, keeping on top of the numbers game is all too familiar. Now I, like others, face borderline high numbers for cholesterol and blood pressure, thanks to my type-A mom and, as my doctor calls it, my "stressful lifestyle." Sometimes, two dogs, one cat, and two fish aren't enough to keep your cholesterol and blood pressure normal.

Instead of turning to heart medications, I've taken the alternative route. I've upped my exercise (swimming and riding a stationary bike), plus you'll find chamomile tea, music, and talking to friends on my daily agenda. But trying to win the battle against the potential for developing heart disease, especially as an aging boomer who also now has less estrogen, is a challenge.

But the good news is, olive oil may be a heart-healthy companion to put in the arsenal against heart disease. In fact, researchers for the U.S. Food and Drug Administration believe olive oil can lower your risk for developing heart disease.

THE "GOOD" FATS

Several years ago, when I interviewed Dr. Artemis P. Simopoulos, author of *The Omega Diet* (HarperCollins, 1998), she told me that there are two kinds of essential fats (EFAs), omega-6 and omega-3. The problem: The American diet contains more omega-6 fatty acids (found in foods such as mayonnaise and salad dressing) than omega-3s. This imbalance makes us more prone to heart disease.

At the time, I wasn't excited about this information, nor did I truly understand it. Today, I realize that this doctor knew what she was talking about, and now I get it. Perhaps, I'm more interested because of the age thing. I realize that if I don't find the delicate balance of EFAs, I may end up taking prescription heart medications, or worse.

SuperFoods Rx author Steven Pratt, M.D., notes in his book that the best balance of omega-6 to omega-3 is somewhere between 1 to 1 and 4 to 1. "Unfortunately, the typical Western diet contains fourteen to twenty-five times more omega-6 than omega-3 fatty acids," he notes. "Too much omega-6 (the oil that dominates our typical diet) promotes an inflammatory state, which in turn increases your risk for blood clots and narrowing of blood vessels."[2]

But the consensus is that the jury is still out about how much omega-3 versus omega-6 you should incorporate in your daily menu. Olive oil, a "good," monounsaturated fat, contains both omega-3 and omega-6 fatty acids.

Dr. Simopoulos offered hope. She told me that we can eat foods that contain the "good" essential fatty acids such as omega-3—found in eggs, fish, and olive oil—along with vegetables, fruits, and legumes. Eating these foods, as do heart healthy people who follow the Mediterranean diet, whether in the European countries or in America, can protect the heart by raising the antioxidant levels, reducing the risk of blood clots, and normalizing blood pressure and heartbeat. Countless people around the world, like you and me, can do the same—begin to balance the EFAs in our diet.

The following heart-healthy tips are from Dr. Simopoulos. Her advice, which I included in my book *Doctors' Orders,* was on target because these helpful hints back up the Mediterranean diet.

- *Enrich your diet with omega-3 fatty acids.* Eat fatty fish, such as salmon two or more times a week.
- *Use olive oil or canola oil as your primary oil.* Canola oil provides monounsaturated fatty acids and LNA, the plant form of omega-3 fatty acids; olive oil has life-enhancing properties.
- *Eat seven or more servings of fruits and vegetables daily.* People in the Mediterranean countries consume plenty of fresh produce, and have enjoyed good health due to the disease-fighting antioxidant benefits.
- *Eat more peas, beans, and nuts.* They are free of saturated fat and cholesterol.
- *Eat less saturated fat and cholesterol.* Both of these increase the risk of heart disease.
- *Avoid oils high in the omega-6 fatty acids.* These include corn oil, safflower oil, peanut oil, soybean oil, sunflower seed oil, cottonseed oil, mayonnaise, and salad dressing.
- *Avoid trans fatty acids.* If you see "partially hydrogenated" on a food label, forgo the product. These substances are often found in baked goods and snack foods.

OLIVE OIL AND BLOOD PRESSURE

For years, I've been writing about the Mediterranean diet, as well as abiding by it myself. In a nutshell, you can have your fat and lower your blood pressure, too, if you eat like they do in Greece and southern Italy, according to medical experts. For instance, if you replace some of the saturated fat, like butter and cheese, in your diet with extra virgin olive oil, you may be able to lower your blood pressure or even cut down on your blood pressure medicine or stop taking it altogether, according to the editors of *The Folk Remedy Encyclopedia.*[3]

The editors add, "But according to the American Institute of Cancer Research olive oil is only a small part of healthy eating in that part of the world." Again, it's the combination of eating little red meat and processed foods, eating more fish and vegetables, and drinking a little red wine that makes the diet healthful—not just one ingredient. It's the total diet and lifestyle package that may help keep blood pressure numbers normal—not just olive oil.[4]

Research shows, too, that a Mediterranean diet, which is similar to the Dietary Approaches to Stop Hypertension (DASH) diet, is linked with both systolic (the top number, which describes the heart's force) and diastolic (the bottom number, which describes the tension between the heartbeats) blood pressure. Olive oil may make as much of a difference as fruits and vegetables in getting a grip on the blood pressure.

And chances are, if you have high blood pressure, you may have high cholesterol, too.

OLIVE OIL AND CHOLESTEROL

Did you know that saturated fat is the main unhealthy culprit in high blood cholesterol? In adults, total cholesterol levels of 240 milligrams per deciliter or higher are considered high risk, and levels from 200 to 239 milligrams per deciliter are considered borderline high risk, according to the AHA.

A middle-aged married couple in Osterville, Massachusetts, told me they are devout users of olive oil—and it seems they are reaping the rewards. C. L. Fornari, aka "The Garden Lady," says, "Both my husband and I have high levels of HDL or 'good' cholesterol, and we are convinced that the amount of olive oil we eat is a major reason for those high levels of HDL." And yes, Fornari is aware that olive oil is rich in disease-fighting polyphenols, which are believed to help control cholesterol levels and lower the risk of heart disease. She adds, "Dan and I use the freshest, full-flavored oils for salads and bread. We use other cold-pressed, virgin oil for cooking."

Research proves that polyphenols can help you stay heart-healthy. A study was done on olive oil and its effects on the hearts of 200 healthy men between the ages of 20 and 60 at six centers in Spain, Denmark, Finland, Italy, and Germany. In a three-week period, the men took a tablespoon of three different olive oils (they varied in phenolic content). The findings: All three of the olive oils raised the "good" cholesterol, lowered the total cholesterol, and lowered triglycerides. The results

proved that the polyphenols in the monounsaturated fatty acid benefits the HDL cholesterol and may lower the risk of developing other
heart problems.[5]

The ADA recommends staying clear of the following saturated fats:

- Foods from animals—beef, beef fat, veal, lamb, pork, lard, poultry,
  butter, cream, milk, and cheeses and other dairy products made
  from whole milk
- Foods from plants—coconut oil, palm oil and palm kernel oil
  (often called tropical oils), and cocoa butter

OLIVE OIL AND BLOOD SUGAR

So, if olive oil can help reduce the risk of developing heart disease,
what can it do about diabetes, especially type 2 diabetes (the non-
insulin type that can be controlled with lifestyle changes and, if necessary, medication)? Yes, the liquid gold comes to the rescue again.

Studies show that olive oil as used in the Mediterranean diet may
help reduce the risk of developing metabolic syndrome—a cluster of
conditions that increase the odds of heart attacks, stroke, and diabetes—which is becoming all too common in baby boomers. If you
have high blood sugar, this is a sign that you may have type 2 diabetes.

A study was conducted at a university hospital in Italy. People with
metabolic syndrome (99 men and 81 women) followed a Mediterranean-
style diet and were taught how to increase their daily intake of whole
grains, fruits, vegetables, nuts, and olive oil.

The results: In two years, researchers found that the Mediterranean
diet group lowered their weight, blood pressure, total cholesterol
(while boosting their "good" HDL cholesterol), triglycerides, glucose,
and insulin. The authors believe that the Mediterranean-style diet
might be a key in fighting metabolic syndrome, an age-related problem that is hitting home in America for both boomers and seniors.[6]

The AHA recommends:

- Further reducing saturated and trans fatty acids in the diet
- Minimizing intake of food and beverages with added sugars

- Emphasizing physical activity and weight control
- Eating a diet rich in vegetables, fruits, and whole-grain foods
- Avoiding tobacco
- Achieving and maintaining healthy cholesterol, blood pressure, and glucose levels

TAKE FATS TO HEART

Trans fats are a hot topic because these hydrogenated fats found in processed foods can be harmful to your heart. According to the AHA, some researchers believe they raise cholesterol levels more than saturated fats do. Plus, trans fats also can up "bad" LDL cholesterol and lower "good" HDL cholesterol when used instead of healthy oils such as olive oil. By switching to heart-healthy oils, you may lower your risk of developing heart disease—high blood pressure, high cholesterol, and diabetes.

The AHA recommends that you:

- Limit your intake of saturated fat to less than 7 percent of your total calories if you are healthy and over the age of 2
- Limit your trans fat to less than 1 percent of your total calories
- Limit your total fat intake to 25 to 35 percent of your total calories
- Get your remaining fat intake from sources of monounsaturated and polyunsaturated fats such as vegetable oils, nuts, seeds, and fish

In addition, did you know that your dentist may be able to predict if you are prone to heart disease? Poor dental hygiene, according to medical experts, can be linked to cardiovascular disease, strokes, and infections. So, while you put olive oil in your daily menu, don't forget to keep your regular dental appointments, too.

As baby boomers and seniors cope with keeping their cholesterol, blood pressure, triglycerides, and blood sugar levels in check, let's take a look at olive oil and its promise to help you lose unwanted body fat and maintain your weight.

The Golden Secrets to Remember

✓ Finding a delicate balance of omega-3s and omega-6s can help you prevent heart disease.

✓ Incorporate more omega-3s—eggs, fish, and olive oil—into your diet to get your essential fatty acids.

✓ Stay clear of oils high in omega-6s—such as salad dressing and mayonnaise. Opt for red wine vinegar and olive oil.

✓ While olive oil may help to lower your blood pressure, don't forget to lose the processed foods and add fish and vegetables to your diet menu.

✓ If your LDL cholesterol is 100 milligrams per deciliter or greater, lower your eating plan to 25 to 35 percent calories from fat. Monitor your saturated fat and dietary cholesterol intake.

✓ To prevent or control type 2 diabetes, cut saturated fats and foods with added sugars from your diet. Plus, focus on regular exercise, and keep your weight in check.

✓ Stay clear of artery-clogging trans fats, found in processed and fried foods. (Read the product label or ask the fast-food chain what type of oil they use.)

11

The Olive Oil Diet

There's probably no food choice you'll make that does more for your health and weight loss efforts than olive oil.

—Connie Peraglier, R.D.[1]

People with high blood pressure and high cholesterol sometimes struggle with tipping the scale—but not always. You can be at your ideal weight and yet have blood pressure higher than 120/80—like me (last night it was 129/72, thanks to a healthful diet and exercise). Blame it on your genes (or the demanding dog), which can play a role in heart disease, and obesity, too.

If you're overweight, keep in mind body fat can attract heart-related diseases like a magnet. The good news is, olive oil may help you to take it off.

Eric Armstrong of Mountain View, California, publisher of TreeLight. com/Health, a Web site devoted to nutrition and fitness, vows that olive oil helps him stave off hunger pangs and boosts his energy—two keys to maintaining your ideal weight.

"I found that building a diet around olive oil helped to suppress hunger and increase energy. Taking it by itself was most effective, but I found it difficult to digest—so I began dipping my bread in it, along with vinegar, as is the custom in Europe. I also put a couple of table-spoons on my cereal in the morning, as part of a dairy-free milk substitute I make myself. It definitely adds to my energy throughout the day," he says.

Indeed, olive oil can suppress your appetite, and perhaps it does just that in Italian-style meals, which include dipping bread into olive oil before beginning the entrée. Keep in mind, however, that while extra virgin olive oil is rich in good-for-you polyphenols, too much of anything can be bad. And yes, that includes olive oil. Remember, it has calories—120 per tablespoon and 14 whopping grams of fat. But, that doesn't stop some people from indulging in the liquid gold by the tablespoon straight from the bottle on a daily basis to lose pounds.

FROM OLIVE OIL TO SHANGRI-LA

Meet Dr. Seth Roberts. Several years ago, he pondered why most diets fail. He decided to be a human rat and used sugar water and extra light olive oil to drop unwanted pounds. When I interviewed the soft-spoken man, he discussed his weight-loss antics.

Back in 2000, Roberts decided to diet because he wanted to be thinner for his 5 foot 11 inch frame. It took him about three months to lose 40 pounds by incorporating fructose water into his diet. He claims that weight is regulated by a "set point." If your weight is below your set point, hunger sets in and you'll want to eat more to feel more satisfied. Roberts believes you can tweak that set point by eating a food that is without flavor—you'll eat less. In fact, Dr. Roberts ended up writing a bestseller, *The Shangri-La Diet: The No Hunger Eat Anything Weight-Loss Plan* (Putnam, 2006) about his experience.

Later, he used extra light olive oil to maintain his weight loss. The idea to take a tablespoon of olive oil—light or not—is a bit hard for me to swallow. But the good professor of psychology at the University of California at Berkeley assured me that it isn't bad at all.

In his book, he writes that a friend told him about "a type of olive, called extra-light" that is bland—no flavor. He notes, "My friend understood that my theory predicted that the most potent weight-loss foods provided calories without flavor. Fructose water did this because of a special wrinkle: sweetness didn't count. ELOO was another way. According to my theory, 100 calories of ELOO should have the same effect as the 100 calories of fructose water."[2]

And it did. But the extra light olive oil also "took less time," according to Dr. Roberts. "No preparation was needed, unlike sugar water." So, it's this olive oil taken daily—just a few spoonfuls daily—that helped the doctor maintain his weight loss. At 5 feet 11 inches, he had lost 40 pounds; and these days, he admitted, he has maintained his weight of a 30-pound weight loss—170 pounds—and gives credit to both the fructose water and the olive oil. "For a few years, I drank only ELOO and didn't use fructose water," he writes. Then, he added the fructose water back in because "it is pleasant."[3]

Also, during our first interview, he told me (and he writes in his book) that he continues to use both—extra light olive oil or some other flavorless oil at home, sucrose water when he's away from home. He doesn't use measured amounts either. If he has packed on a few pounds, he will drink more. If he is too "thin," he will drink less.

These days, Roberts is experimenting once again, and this time it's with walnut oil (1 tablespoon) and flaxseed oil (2 tablespoons) daily. "I am still trying to determine the optimum type and amount of oil but I am sure I will continue forever because of the weight and health benefits."

Speaking of different diets, as a former diet and nutrition columnist for *Woman's World* magazine, I used to write about every diet imaginable, from the cabbage soup diet to high-protein diets.

EAT FAT TO LOSE FAT

It's funny, but as I wrote about paring pounds, I continued to eat the Mediterranean diet type of foods—vegetables, fruits, whole grains, even pizza—and I maintained my 122 pounds through it all. Despite the fact that I didn't have a weight problem, I once again was faced with progressive medical doctors discussing "good" fats with me.

I interviewed Dr. Barry Sears, for example, who wrote *Enter the Zone*. He told me that it was important to add the right amount of fat to your diet. Yes, fat!

"I know it's shocking," Dr. Sears said, "but you have to eat fat in order to lose fat. You have to stop thinking of food in terms of calories and fat grams alone and start thinking of it as a mechanism for controlling the flow of hormones."

The fact is, fats and proteins trigger the release of hormones that neutralize the effect of insulin released by carbohydrates. So, adding more fat and protein to your diet means you'll actually store less fat.

But you don't want to load up on saturated fat, the artery-clogging fat found mainly in animal products. You want to avoid these fats because they tend to raise insulin levels, which will defeat your fat-burning goal. In Chapter 8, "More Healing Oils," I discuss the oils that are good for you. It's these same oils that can help you to fight fat forever.

I also interviewed nutritionists Gene and Joyce Daoust, who taught me about "good" fats, too. They told me unsaturated fat (vegetable oils like safflower oil, sunflower oil, and corn oil) and monounsaturated fat (olive oil, canola oil, olives, macadamia nuts, and avocados) are good for you and can help you to burn fat.

Here are some important facts I learned about eating "good" fat:

- It boosts your energy.
- It triggers the release of CCK, a hormone that signals your brain that you're full and should stop eating.
- It contains fat-soluble compounds to help metabolize fat-soluble vitamins A, D, E, and K.
- It contains omega-3 and omega-6 fatty acids (found in fatty fishes, such as tuna), which are essential for fat metabolism.
- It helps slow down the rate of carbohydrate absorption into the bloodstream and helps to lower the rate of insulin secretion.

USE YOUR FAT BUDGET

So, we do need some fat. The consensus is to consume about 40 to 60 grams per day. Also, do not deprive yourself of good-for-you fatty foods—some with olive oil, others without.

Favorite Food	"Good" Fats	Fat Grams
Pizza	Order vegetable toppings, and hold the meat and extra cheese; drizzle olive oil on top; and order a dark green side salad with vegetables.	5 grams per slice
Peanut butter	A rich spread high in fat, but it's mainly monounsaturated and polyunsaturated fats,	8 grams per tablespoon

Favorite Food	"Good" Fats	Fat Grams
	which are healthier for your heart than saturated fat.	
Eggs	Even though egg yolks contain fat, they also contain vitamins A, B, D, and E.	6 grams per egg
Avocados	High in fat, but most of it is monounsaturated, which tends to improve cholesterol and protect rather than clog arteries.	8 grams per fruit
Almonds	"Almonds are probably the best all-around nut. Most of the fats of the almond are polyunsaturated and high in linoleic acid, our main essential oil," notes Elson Haas, M.D., author of *Staying Healthy with Nutrition* (Celestial Arts, 2006).	5.4 grams per 10 nuts

THE SKINNY ON TRANS FATS

The good news is that "trans fats" is becoming a household word. You can pick up a food item and read the label to see if it contains trans fats—those bad-for-you partially hydrogenated vegetable oils found in packaged, processed foods. It's lurking inside such items as pastries, pies, cookies, cakes, muffins, margarine, and vegetable shortening.

Thanks to the FDA guidelines of January 1, 2006, the labeling of foods includes the amount of trans fats in each product. The glitch is that food manufacturers are hesitant to stop using trans fats, since this ingredient is less costly than healthier oils such as olive oil—and it helps preserve products' shelf life. Worse, many of these fatty foods containing these fats claim to be trans fat–free.

A good way to decode foods for their trans fat content is to check the ingredients list. If you see the words "partially hydrogenated oils," "hydrogenated oils," or "vegetable shortening," stay clear. These are red flags and—nice words for a "bad" fat.

This can get tricky. For instance, I purchased a box of dark chocolate brownie mix. I wanted to add olive oil to see if it worked and tasted good. The food label read, "Trans fat 0 g," but it also included the words "partially hydrogenated soybean and/or cottonseed oil."

Confused and hesitant to bake my healthful brownies, I contacted Marisa Moore, R.D., American Dietetic Association spokesperson based in Atlanta, Georgia. She told me, "According to the US Food and Drug Administration (FDA) guidelines, trans fat does not have to be listed if the total fat in a product is less than 0.5 grams per serving and no claims are made about fat, fatty acids and cholesterol content."

In addition, Moore says, "If trans fats per serving equals 0.5 grams or less, manufacturers are allowed to list the trans fat as 0 (zero) on the label. Therefore, you may find products that list 0 grams trans fat on the label, while 'partially hydrogenated vegetable oil' appears in the ingredient list."

Rather than play the game of seeing how far down the list of ingredients trans fats may be, it's safer to change your game plan of buying food and cooking it. The best advice: If you follow the Mediterranean Diet—vegetables, fruits, grains, fish, legumes, and olive oil—you won't have to decipher packaged goods. You will be eating fresh foods, and this will help you to fight fat, and to lower your risk of developing age-related diseases that are linked to body fat, too.

An easy-to-remember rule is: Limit your intake of trans fats to no more than 1 percent of your total calories. On a 2,000-calorie diet, that equals 2 grams per day. "It's important to seek products that are trans fat free and also low in saturated fat," says Moore. That way, you can achieve a trim, healthy body.

The American Heart Association also recommends that you follow these do's and don'ts to help slash trans fats:

Do	Don't
Use olive oil and canola oil.	Use foods made with hydrogenated or saturated fat.
Use margarine as a substitute for butter.	Use hard stick forms of butter.
Use margarine that contains no more than 2 grams of saturated	Eat foods that contain trans fats, which include french fries, dough-

Do	Don't
fat per tablespoon and that lists liquid vegetable oil as the first ingredient.	nuts, cookies, and crackers. Eat foods that contain saturated fat, and you won't consume a lot of trans fats.
Avoid commercially fried foods and commercially baked goods.	Eat foods labeled "trans fat free," and look for the words "partially hydrogenated" as a red flag.

NEVER DIET AGAIN

You really don't have to deprive yourself to lose pounds or maintain your weight. It's all about incorporating healthful eating habits into your lifestyle. For instance, when I go to a sandwich outlet, I order whole wheat bread, extra tomatoes, lettuce, green bell peppers, one piece of swiss chesse, olive oil, and vinegar. And now, I also ask for avocado and olives.

Speaking of olives . . . Recently, I ordered a vegetarian pizza. Usually, I order the normal tomato sauce, spinach, and mushrooms. This time, however, I overheard the man who took my order say "basil" and "olive oil." I quickly inquired, since I had no clue they offered a pesto sauce with these two items. So, I ordered the green sauce with spinach, tomatoes, and olives. Do you see how you can treat yourself to full-fat foods and still eat healthy as well as not pack on unwanted pounds? What's more, if time allows, you can whip up your own pizza and use pesto sauce.

Basil and Spinach Pesto with Walnuts

❖ ❖ ❖

1 bunch fresh spinach
1 bunch basil
5 cloves garlic
¾ cup Spectrum Naturals Tuscan
    Style Extra Virgin Olive Oil

¼ cup toasted walnuts
¼ cup Parmesan cheese

In a blender, combine half the greens and all of the garlic. Add half of the oil and blend until pureed. Add the rest of the greens, a handful at a time, adding more oil as needed. Add the walnuts and cheese, and continue to puree. Season with salt and pepper. Pesto can be stored covered in the refrigerator for two weeks or frozen for up to six months. Makes approximately 1½ cups.

(*Source:* Chef Gary Jenanyan)

Once you realize that you can eat food and have your pizza, too, you'll get a handle on your weight. But then, while maintaining your ideal weight, there's the aging factor, which affects more than body fat and pounds. In the next chapter, I will discuss why olive oil is getting a good reputation around the world for turning back the clock.

THE GOLDEN SECRETS TO REMEMBER

✓ Olive oil can help to suppress your appetite. Go ahead—drizzle it on bread the way Europeans do before a meal . . .

✓ . . . But don't overdo a good thing. Olive oil is a fat and does have 120 calories per tablespoon.

✓ Extra light olive oil, which is without flavor, may help you to maintain your weight, or "set point."

✓ Eating "good" fats can give you energy, stop you from overeating, help your body metabolize the fat-soluble vitamins, and provide essential fatty acids.

✓ Savor a moderate amount of fatty foods such as pizza and eggs because these favorites contain "good" fats and other nutrients.

✓ Learn how to decode the ingredients lists of food products, which often call trans fats "partially hydrogenated oils," "hydrogenated oils," or "vegetable oils." Then run, not walk, away from these foods.

✓ To get a trim body, limit your intake of trans fats to no more than 1 percent of your total calories.

Antiaging Wonder Food

Italians . . . seemed to never die. They eat olive oil
all day long . . . and that's what does it.
—William Kennedy[1]

One morning after I finished my breakfast of fruit and oatmeal, I pondered, "Why is Japan, not Greece, ranked number-one for longevity?" I quickly called my go-to person, *The Omega Diet* author Artemis P. Simopoulos, M.D., and asked her, "Why aren't the Europeans ranked as having the longest life span? What about the Mediterranean diet?"

She told me that the Cretes did have the longest life span, as well as the lowest rates of heart disease and cancer, thanks to eating antioxidant-rich foods. But lately, they have been replacing these good foods with the high-fat and processed foods of the Western diet, much like the traditional Hawaiians, whom I wrote about several years ago. Fast food is cheaper and faster, but the numbers show that eating it also leads to a shorter life.

Other nutritionists and medical doctors agree. People in the European countries as well as in America are spending less time cooking in the kitchen and more time eating at fast-food chains and restaurants, which boast unhealthy fats. Still, on the upside, more chefs and food outlets know that Mediterranean fare is healthy and so are offering the anti-oxidant-rich antiaging foods, including heart-healthy oils such as canola and olive oil.

Can Olive Oil Turn Back the Clock?

Recently, I took one of those online "Real Age" tests (www.realage. com/). Since I've been tagged a health and fitness expert, you would think that I'd pass the self-quiz with flying colors, right? Well, not exactly. My real age was 52.1, which was 2.2 years less than my calendar age of 54.2. While I wasn't thrilled, I realized it could be worse. Jim Berkland, my health-savvy friend who is in his seventies, told me he took a similar test and his results were that he had expired.

To me, the test results seemed on target. But I got a second opinion from Marisa Moore, R.D, American Dietetic Association spokesperson. She gave me the low-down on my dietary needs, based upon my test evaluation and recommendations. It's as easy as 1-2-3.

1   **More Vitamin E:** The test results suggested I up my intake of vitamin E. Well, I looked at my "complete multi-vitamin-mineral" supplement. It supplies 60 international units of vitamin E, or 20 percent of my daily requirement. Moore says, "Based on the Dietary Reference Intakes (DRIs), healthy adult women and men should aim for 15 mg vitamin E per day. The recommendation is the same for males and females greater than 14 years old." Your best food sources are walnut oil, soybean oil, olive oil, peanut butter, and wheat germ.

2   **More Essential Fatty Acids:** Then, the test analysis hit me in the belly because I prefer to be a vegan—a strict one most of the time. It was recommended that I add fish or other sources of omega-3 fatty acids to my diet at least several times a week.

   Moore says, "Aim for 1–2grams of omega-3 fatty acids per day. This is ideal to help reduce LDL (bad) cholesterol and to help with brain development. It's best to get your omega-3s from food." So, again, I now have albacore tuna in my pantry; I also purchase fresh salmon. But, I confess I don't like fish as much as I did as a kid. Also, those little signs about mercury toxins that stare at me while I stand in line to purchase fresh fish at the supermarket are a bit scary. The omega-3s are found in more than just salmon and tuna.

   "Omega-3 fatty acids are polyunsaturated fats found mostly in seafood. Good sources include fatty, cold-water fish such as mackerel, halibut and herring. Flaxseeds, flax oil and walnuts also contain omega-3 fatty acids, and small amounts are found in soybean and canola oils. They have a protective effect by reducing blood clot formation, reducing triglyceride levels and may be important in your diet to help prevent cardiovascular disease. Aim for 2 servings of fish per week," explains Moore.

Immediately, I purchased those all-natural doggie treats (with canola oil) for my two pooches. I include a canola oil–based spread for old time's sake. Walnuts I can do.

3 **More Unsaturated Fat:** The test results also noted that I should eat more unsaturated fat without increasing my consumption of saturated fat. Worse, because I evidently am eating less than the average amount of unsaturated fats, my biological age may be slightly older. "How could this be?" I pondered. "I am an olive oil book author."

Moore says, "Olive oil is a great way to increase your intake of heart healthy fats. You can also use olive oil to make salad dressings, drizzle on grilled or roasted vegetables, in marinades and sautés." Plus, she adds, "Olive oil is a great source of monounsaturated fats while soybean and corn oil are polyunsaturated fats. Both fats may help lower your blood cholesterol when used in place of saturated fats in your diet." Ironically, I know this now, but I guess it's a task to practice what you preach.

I had thought that my borderline high blood pressure and cholesterol were due to genes, not my diet. Yes, until recently, I used butter on my baked potatoes and pastas. It's true, I have eaten those big bran and pumpkin muffins and extra large bagels from bakeries—which use unhealthy fats. This test—and Moore's personal comments—taught me that while I thought I was on the "good"-fats track, there is more I can do—starting with incorporating olive oil, vitamin E, and fish in my daily diet. But that's not all . . .

HEALTH INSURANCE AND OLIVE OIL

While that Real Age test was a wake-up call, a letter from my health insurance company got me on my feet and to the telephone. "Why are you raising my monthly rate twenty-five percent?" I asked. "I am in Tier One—that's a category where the healthy people are put." The young man said it was because of my *age*. Oh my, the age factor again. He told me that as people age, they begin to have health problems. Worse, when I hit the big 55, my rates will soar even higher whether I stay healthy or not.

So, rather than cancel my health insurance, I decided it's worth it to have peace of mind in case an age-related disease hits me, but . . . That rate increase has gotten me onto a preventive health care plan on which I follow the Real Age experts' recommendations—up the "good" fats and lose the "bad" fats. After all, this advice, which I include in this book, may stave off high blood pressure, high cholesterol, diabetes, cancer, and more. But let's face it, olive oil isn't the only food that will save me from growing older faster.

THE FOUNTAIN OF OIL AND VINEGAR

I often tout the antiaging potential of both red wine and balsamic vinegars. Why? Researchers I interviewed several years ago said there's a possibility that vinegar contains resveratrol just like heart-healthy red wine and grape juice. Well, in 1999 *and* 2006, Dr. LeRoy Creasy analyzed a cheap red wine vinegar, and both times, he claims, he didn't find any resveratrol. But the question remains, if he used a high-quality vinegar, would it make a difference?

Still, even if red wine and balsamic vinegars contain only disease-fighting polyphenols (and we know they do), some foods such as blueberries, plums, peanuts, and red wine—all part of the Mediterranean diet—do indeed contain resveratrol.

So, teaming these antiaging foods with olive oil may help people around the globe—not just in the Mediterranean basin—to lose body fat and stall age-related diseases. These resveratrol-rich foods combined with other nutrient-rich "superfoods" that contain other disease-fighting compounds can help people fight the aging process and live a longer, healthier life.

Speaking of turning back the clock, I started noticing articles online about challenges of aging. Now, I wrote about all of those topics in my book *Doctors' Orders*. However, when I am hit with Real Age test results and told I need to pay higher health insurance rates, you can bet that I'm going to get my aging woes in a row.

DEFYING AGING WITH OLIVE OIL

Arthritis

The Aging Factor: As we age, our joints begin to degenerate. According to the Arthritis Foundation, osteoarthritis affects nearly 21 million Americans, mostly after age 45; women are more commonly affected than men.

It's Personal: In my fifties, I don't have arthritis yet, but I know people who do have aches and pains. While a heating pad does the trick for me after I shovel snow or overdo it on the bike or using hand weights, it doesn't mean that I am immune to arthritis woes. A friend of mine who is my age does have arthritis, in her hip. A neighbor who is 70 has osteoarthritis and is nearly bedridden. And, I can't forget how my late beloved Brittany, Dylan, suffered from arthritis—a problem I never thought would affect a 40-pound dog. But to watch him not be able to jump up into the car or onto the bed was enough to make me see how stiff joints are not fun.

Olive Oil + Rx: While olive oil can be beneficial, omega-3 oils are also important for the lubrication of joints. They reduce prostaglandins. Also, rheumatologists will tell you that staying physically active (like recommended in the Mediterranean lifestyle) is another way to shake the pain of stiff joints.

Cancer

The Aging Factor: The longer we live, the greater are our odds of facing cancer—when free radical molecules in the body cause normal cells to grow and divide in an out-of-control manner.

It's Personal: The big C is frightening to everyone (at any age). My father died of liver cancer. As a DES daughter (DES is a synthetic estrogen that was given to about 4.8 million women in the United States between 1938 and 1971, and has been linked to a rare from of cancer in their daughters and sons), when I have regular Pap smears, I can't forget that I am at a higher risk for developing cervical cancer. Again, as we age, cancer becomes a more likely scenario, whether it is skin cancer or breast cancer—it can affect all of us. Nobody is immune—not me, you, or even our pets.

Olive Oil + Rx: Research continues to show that olive oil may help prevent cancers because of its polyphenols. The American Cancer Society stands by its five to nine servings of vegetables and fruits per day, which may also lower your risk of developing cancer, which increases with age. And, of course, olive oil can help add flavor to fresh produce.

Heart Disease

The Aging Factor: Medical doctors will tell you that the older you get, the more your risks of high cholesterol and high blood pressure go up.

It's Personal: My mother had high blood pressure. I remember that in her thirties, she even had a cardiologist. But, it was her unhealthy lifestyle (smoking, drinking, and stress) that certainly fueled her heart problems. While I have never smoked or had a drop of alcohol, I did inherit her type-A personality, which is linked to heart disease.

Olive Oil + Rx: Research shows that olive oil can help lower the risk of developing heart disease. But, it is the Mediterranean diet and lifestyle (including regular exercise) that can help stave off heart problems. So, remember that fish, whole grains, fruits, vegetables, and getting physical every day along with consuming olive oil may keep you heart-healthy for years. And, learning how to chill is part of the anti–heart disease plan.

Obesity

The Aging Factor: Middle-age spread affects both women and men, thanks to changing hormones and a slower metabolism. Often, body fat ends up on the belly, and this can create health woes from heart disease to diabetes.

It's Personal: As a former hippie, I recall how it was stylish to be thin like models. In my teens, I struggled with bulimia and anorexia.. We didn't have names for these eating disorders then, nor were there support groups. I ended up going back to college, and once I had a new life, I learned that healthful food was my friend and overeating or not eating was my enemy.

Olive Oil + Rx: Anecdotal evidence shows that olive oil can suppress the appetite. The older you get, the more you want to stay physically active, to burn off your calories instead of storing body fat. Teaming olive oil with fat-burning foods such as vegetables, whole grains, and fish may also help you keep satisfied, as well as maintain a lean body throughout your life span.

Osteoporosis

The Aging Factor: The "brittle bone" disease can strike at any age. Osteoporosis, the loss of bone density, is often thought of as an older person's disease—but it can strike as early as the thirties, forties, and fifties. But note, the chances of bone loss increase as you age, because your bones become less dense and weaker.

It's Personal: Years ago, I had a neighbor, Ruth, 69, who was a retired widow. I used to watch her walk to the grocery store. It was a sight to see because she had become disfigured with a "dowager's hump." Think of the wicked witch in the *Wizard of Oz*. This image is frightening to many people, like me, who are at risk. As we age, estrogen plummets, especially after menopause, and the incidence of bone loss rises. Women are about four times more apt to develop bone loss. Caucasian (like me) and Asian women are more likely to develop bone loss. Small-boned people—again, women (like me)—are at greater risk.

Olive Oil + Rx: Olive oil solo may help beat bone loss. However, other fatty acids—the "good" fats—also play various roles in bone structure, function, and development. The fact is, fats are necessary for good calcium metabolism and are essential components of cartilage and bone. Best sources: olive oil, fish oil, and flaxseed oil.

Teeth

The Aging Factor: Baby boomers and seniors these days can and do have their own teeth. Dentures are the last resort. In the twenty-first century, we have modern dentistry, from crowns to dental implants, that help us preserve our own smile, unlike our parents in the twentieth century.

It's Personal: Since I was a teenager, I have been on a healthy teeth campaign. I wore braces. I endured cavities and fillings. In my twenties, I had a crown, and then one day, a root canal. Today, while I still have my own teeth—like the majority of boomers and seniors who practice good dental hygiene—I know that I have to floss and brush daily, see the dentist twice a year (at least), and use one of those sonic toothbrushes to keep gingivitis and periodontal disease at bay.

Olive Oil + Rx: Perhaps using a water-and-olive-oil rinse to protect your teeth if you grind at night will help keep your pearly whites in good condition. But a healthful diet, such as the Mediterranean eating plan (with minimal sweets), drinking six to eight 8-ounce glasses of water daily, taking a multi-vitamin-mineral supplement each day, and visiting your dentist as needed are also musts to keep your teeth forever young.

Vision

The Aging Factor: Glaucoma and macular degeneration are age-related problems. Both can lead to blindness. Plus, with an increased longevity and decreased good nutrition, good eyesight may not be in the cards.

It's Personal: Eyesight is a precious thing that we take for granted until we reach our forties. Then, before we know it, we need reading glasses for the small print in newspapers and on food labels. Later, the glasses are must-haves for the computer. Also, macular degeneration is a frightening eye problem that I have witnessed in two friends. Both are legally blind.

Olive Oil + Rx: Magnesium-rich foods can help prevent glaucoma and improve blood circulation, according to ophthalmologist Robert Abel Jr., M.D., of Wilmington, Delaware. Antioxidant-rich foods (which taste better with olive oil) and vitamin E–rich oils like soybean oil, corn oil, peanut oil, safflower oil, and sesame oil can help protect against macular degeneration, notes Charles Kroll, an optometrist in Chicago, Illinois. These foods can taste better with olive oil—which also contains antioxidant vitamin E.

As I communicate with other aging boomers and seniors, I realize that aging is not fun. However, if we can help ourselves age gracefully and maintain our health, I feel that while it is a challenge, it doesn't have to be the end of our world as we know it.

In Part 5, "Olive Oil Home Remedies," you'll discover some amazing ways to use olive oil to help you feel better and look great—whether it's for moisturizing your skin from head to toe or keeping your companion animals forever younger, too.

THE GOLDEN SECRETS TO REMEMBER

✓ You can take years off your biological age by changing your diet and lifestyle—and olive oil can play a part.
✓ As health insurance rates go up, if you increase the "good" fats and lose the "bad" fats, you can lower your risk of developing age-related diseases.
✓ Teaming antioxidant-rich red wine and balsamic vinegars with Mediterranean diet foods that are rich in resveratrol may help you lose body fat as well as win the aging game.
✓ Omega-3 oils can help stave off the aches and pains of arthritis as you age.
✓ Polyphenol-rich olive oil may help to lower your risk of developing age-related cancers.
✓ Heart-healthy olive oil can help you maintain healthy blood pressure, cholesterol, and blood sugar numbers, which will beat heart disease and diabetes.
✓ Research proves olive oil can help you maintain your weight (a

problem in aging boomers and seniors) by keeping hunger pangs at bay.

✓ "Good" fats such as olive oil and other fatty acids strengthen bone density, which can help you beat bone loss (at any age).

✓ Olive oil as a protective mouth rinse, as well as a healthful diet and regular dental checkups, can preserve your pearly whites.

PART 5

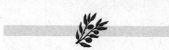

OLIVE OIL HOME REMEDIES

Cures from Your Kitchen

Only the sea itself seems as ancient a part of the region as the olive and its oil, that like no other products of nature, have shaped civilizations from remotest antiquity to the present.
—Lawrence Durrell[1]

On June 26, 2007, I like hundreds of people in South Lake Tahoe, endured enormous stress due to an out of control wildfire. Stress is triggered partly by the sensitivity of our sympathetic system, which jump-starts the fight-or-flight reaction. So when the pressure is on, up go our pulse rate, respiration and muscle tension. The bottom line: I was scared and my companion animals were excited.

Once I realized the fire was too close to home, I chose to flee to escape the smoke inhalation, helicopters, sirens, ash, automated evacuation telephone calls, gridlock due to closed roads, and mass chaos of the Angora Fire.

I grabbed my must-have essentials: two dogs, one cat, a brother (in denial), a pile of clothes, a laptop computer, pet food and supplies, and my purse full of personal items. Once we settled in at a pet-friendly hotel in Reno, Nevada, I realized hour by hour that I didn't have two items I'm used to having for comfort, beauty, and pesky human and pet ailments.

I didn't have extra virgin olive oil (which I use on my skin, feet, hands and hair) nor did I have vinegar for Simon, my dog's sore nose (evidently his was bit by something) and his abraded paws due to the hot asphalt and wet grass during his walks). It hit me. I missed having both oil and vinegar—two universal liquids—for emergencies, like this unforgettable one, because they have so many uses when you are away and back at home.

Chances are, olive oil, canola oil, coconut oil, and other oils—your everyday household products—contain even more extraordinary healing powers that you might not know about. The next time you need a natural remedy for an ailment, check this list first to see if a cure is as close as your kitchen cabinet or pantry.

I'll describe common health ailments and cosmetic problems, from A to Z, and provide at-home healing-oil folk remedies. Some treatments can be used inside and others outside the body. Keep in mind these are based on anecdotal evidence. There are no hard-hitting studies to back up their effectiveness and make it conclusive.

30 AMAZING OIL REMEDIES

Did you know that olive oil (and other oils) is considered one of the most popular folk remedies? Well, if this surprises you, read on, and you'll see why oil remedies are good to have in your home, wherever you live. But note, use common sense, and consult your doctor, before starting any new treatments—folk remedies or not.

1 BEAT BLADDER INFECTIONS Bladder infection coming on? You begin to urinate but feel a burning pain. It may be a bladder infection, also called a urinary tract infection (UTI). Worse, you may feel an urgency to urinate and pain in the lower back and pelvic area. Bacteria can cause bladder infections. Also, the hormonal changes that hit at menopause can trigger UTIs. Some medical experts believe that when estrogen declines, the pH level of the vagina changes and the number of good bacteria declines.

What Oil Remedy to Use: One teaspoon of olive oil and one teaspoon of garlic juice mixed in a glass of warm water. Drink three times a day, preferably before meals. It also may be helpful to drink cranberry juice as a preventative measure.

Why You'll Like It: It's a pain to take time out to go to the doctor. It's also a pain to deal with the side effects that come with the antibiotics commonly used to treat bladder infections.

2 BABY SKIN BURNS Ever accidentally burn yourself while cooking, stoking wood in a fireplace, or drinking a beverage that is just too hot? Like bladder infections, burns can be painful, and the pain can last for a while. Since biblical times, people have turned to the almighty olive and its oil to help heal burns naturally.

What Oil Remedy to Use: Apply extra virgin olive oil on your burn three or four times daily.

Why You'll Like It: Not only is it natural, but olive oil doesn't have a strong medicine smell. Also, its antibiotic effect does the job. If you burn your mouth or lip, olive oil is gentle and edible.

3 BYE-BYE BRUXISM In the twenty-first century, people are preserving their pearly whites throughout their lifetime, unlike in the twentieth century, when dentures were more common. These days, if you brush your teeth and floss regularly, get checkups twice a year, and have dental cleanings as needed, you have a good chance of keeping your smile. And, olive oil may help, too.

"Olive oil has been shown to decrease tooth wear, but only in small studies where it was used to minimize the damage caused by grinding (bruxism). It acted as a lubricant in combination with an acrylic tooth guard," notes California olive oil expert John Deane, M.D.

What Oil Remedy to Use: Before bedtime, rinse your mouth with an emulsion of olive oil and water to decrease plaque (the sticky substance that can create inflammation of the gums or gingivitis).

Why You'll Like It: What's not to like? If this easy, all-natural mouth rinse can help to preserve your teeth, why not give it a go? Plus, some mouthwash rinses are strong and can discolor your teeth temporarily, until you have them professionally cleaned by a dental hygienist.

4 CURE A COUGH Do you have a nagging cough? A tickle in your throat can be more annoying than a skin burn. Often, coughs occur after a cold or are linked to an allergy. The fact is, if you're hacking during the day or night, you (and others around you) have one sentence on the brain: "How can I make that annoying cough go away?"

What Oil Remedy to Use: Take 1 tablespoon of olive oil as needed.

Why You'll Like It: It may be just what you need to help you chase away that cough because it will lubricate a tickle in your throat. A bonus: Olive oil doesn't contain undesirable ingredients (for example, codeine) that commercial syrups do, and it may even taste better than some.

5 CAN CONSTIPATION Speaking of annoyances . . . Feeling irregular? You're hardly alone. Often, a change in climate or travel can wreak havoc on your regularity. Constipation can affect you (at any age). Forget cod liver oil. It doesn't taste very good, and there is a more practical remedy.

What Oil Remedy to Use: Take 1 tablespoon of extra virgin olive oil with vegetables and fruits. Don't forget to enjoy five to nine servings daily.

Why You'll Like It: Olive oil and veggies is an all-natural remedy that works. Increasing your intake of fresh produce, drinking plenty of water—six to eight 8 ounce glasses daily—and getting regular exercise also can help you stay regular.

6 CODDLE CUTICLES Dry cuticles? Many people (at any age), especially those who live in cold climates, suffer from bouts of dry hands and dry cuticles. Worse, if you tear the hanging skin, it can lead to an open cut or wound. If you ignore dry cuticles, you can end up with an infection.

What Oil Remedy to Use: Try applying olive oil directly to your hands and cuticles twice daily. Also, use an olive oil–based soap.

Why You'll Like It: Teaming the two home cures works like a charm. One devout user told me, "I keep a small container of it handy for rubbing into my cuticles. Keeps them super soft and smelling less artificial than most moisturizers on the market these days."

7 EASE AN EARACHE Ears throb? Like a cough or irregular bowel habits, an earache can drive you crazy. I endured an ear infection (due to the cold, dry winter weather). So, I went to the bathroom cabinet to reach for those prescribed eardrops. The date had expired. This time around, it was in the fall, and I knew it was swimmer's ear due to a regular routine of swimming laps at the gym. It was late at night, so I turned to olive oil instead.

What Oil Remedy to Use: Put a few drops of olive oil in the ear canal. Repeat as needed.

Why You'll Like It: For one, if it's a minor earache, olive oil, which is believed to have mild antibiotic properties, can and does get rid of the ache and heal the pain.

8 DUMP DANDRUFF Dry flakes and dry scalp? It can be a pesky cosmetic issue (unlike an ear infection), since dandruff can get out of control. Before you run to the dermatologist, consider using both conditioning olive oil and antibacterial vinegar, which kill the bacteria that is believed to be the cause.

What Oil Remedy to Use: Beauty experts suggest combining both vinegar and olive oil with water. I suggest 2 tablespoons of apple cider vinegar, 2 tablespoons of spring water, and 2 tablespoons of extra virgin olive oil. Mix them together, then massage them into your scalp. Rinse after 20 minutes, and shampoo.

Why You'll Like It: Ever smell dandruff shampoos? Ugh! The unnatural scent and harsh chemicals are enough to make you scream out loud in disgust before handling the toxic-smelling shampoo, let alone putting it on your sacred crown. Opt for a natural oil remedy, and see if it works for you.

9 DISS DIAPER RASH Almost everyone has seen a diaper rash, which is an infant's reddened bottom. There are store-bought remedies, but if you aren't near a store, what to do? Many olive oil experts say olive oil has been used to treat diaper rash in olive-producing countries such as Italy. Antonio gives kudos to his grandmother for her "washed oil" special remedy, which works for both a sunburn and a "baby's inflamed bottom."

What Oil Remedy to Use: Use 2 teaspoons of extra virgin olive oil with 1 teaspoon of water. Shake these two ingredients until you get a pasty emulsion, a sort of cream ready to be spread on your body.

Why You'll Like It: Not only does Antonio validate this remedy, but as a "mom" with three fur children, I can tell you that if there is a natural remedy for an ailment, I will turn to it before using a product with chemicals in it. So, Antonio's grandma's "magic ointment" may make both you and your child or grandchild tickled pink when it clears up the redness on baby.

10 FIX YOUR SORE FEET All of us have had to stand on our feet longer than we would have liked, whether it was to feed a baby with a diaper rash, to wait in line with a baby at the grocery store or airport, or perhaps to take a hike solo for fun. If you have been there, done that, you may have wished for a quick cure to soothe away the pain. Some olive oil fans who believe in its folklore magic also believe it can pamper tired feet.

What Oil Remedy to Use: Try a soak in a pan of warm water. Dilute 3 drops of lavender essential oil, 2 drops of eucalyptus essential oil, and 2 drops of lemon essential oil in 2 teaspoons of olive oil. Add to a footbath.

Why You'll Like It: A relaxing soak can ease the cares of the day, and the olive oil combination relieves foot soreness.

11 FORGET FIBROMYALGIA Want to shake aches and pains in your muscles? If you have tenderness in eleven or more of the eighteen "tender points," which include the back of the neck, lower back, and lateral hips, you may have fibromyalgia. Or, if your tender points don't reach eleven you still may have a flare-up, especially during stressful times, or when cold-weather changes hit.

What Oil Remedy to Use: Eating an antioxidant-rich diet complete with vegetables, fruits, and fish drizzled with olive oil, which has anti-inflammatory properties, may help. Also, try massaging the areas on your body that ache.

Why You'll Like It: If you can get relief from sore, stiff muscles, you will feel more comfortable and will be able to resume normal daily activities.

12 GOOD-BYE GALLBLADDER PROBLEMS It's no secret that obesity is a risk factor for gallstones. Also, if you have cholesterol woes and eat fatty foods, you may be experiencing gallbladder trouble. Your first line of action should be to up your fiber intake, eat a low-fat diet, and lose some unwanted weight. Some natural-cure practitioners tout an olive oil remedy to cleanse excess refined carbs, sugar, and fat.

What Oil Remedy to Use: Try approximately 2 tablespoons of olive oil chased by 1/2 cup grapefruit or lemon juice each morning for one week.

Why You'll Like It: If it works in conjunction with your new gallbladder diet and lifestyle, you may not be haunted by developing gallstones or needing surgery.

13 GOOD RIDDANCE TO GINGIVITIS Puffy gums? Pink toothbrush? Bleeding gums? Welcome to gingivitis—inflammation of the gums. Certainly, regular brushing, flossing, and dental checkups and cleanings are preventative measures. But can olive oil help fight red and swollen gums and stave off periodontal problems, which can lead to tooth loss?

What Oil Remedy to Use: Rinse your mouth with an emulsion of olive oil and water.

Why You'll Like It: According to Dr. Deane, small studies have shown that this olive oil remedy can decrease plaque, the sticky substance that can form into tartar, which only a dental cleaning can remove. If you want to ward off periodontal disease and save your pearly whites, it may be worth a try.

14 HALT HAIR LOSS Both men and women may need to cope with thinning hair, which can be due to many causes, from hormones or genetics to nutritional deficiencies. If you're not getting enough essential fatty acids or vitamins A and E—all components of olive oil—this home cure may help you maintain the strength of your hair.

What Oil Remedy to Use: Take 1 tablespoon of extra virgin olive oil daily or use it in your food, especially foods with essential fatty acids, such as slivered almonds and tuna.

Why You'll Like It: Olive oil incorporated into your diet can help keep your hair nourished and soft. Vitamin A helps keep hair strong, and vitamin E retards the aging of skin cells. But note, if you are a man, you may consider shaving your head, which to many people is attractive. Using olive oil will give the skin on your head a healthful sheen.

15 HANG UP A HANGOVER Killer headache? Ever suffer the day after from drinking too much alcohol? The symptoms can be nasty, including a bad headache, nausea, and sensitivity to light and sound. Rather than deal, it might be easier to try an olive oil cure.

What Oil Remedy to Use: On the Internet, you can find a variety of references to a "prairie cocktail," which is a concoction of olive oil, tomato ketchup, and vinegar.

Why You'll Like It: Well, one desperate gentleman claimed it made him sick. But it is believed that the olive oil cleanses the gallbladder and liver, as well as soothes the tummy.

16 HIT ILLNESS WITH ANTIBACTERIAL HAND SOAP Want to avoid getting sick during the cold and flu season? Since washing your hands often can help stave off contagious illnesses, which usually make the rounds in the fall and winter, a good antibacterial soap can help you. One holiday season, I forgot to buy hand soap. I had to create a quick remedy. I had purchased antibacterial dish soap, but I thought, "This is going to be too harsh on my hands." So, I turned to versatile olive oil.

What Oil Remedy to Use: Pour 3 parts antibacterial dish soap and 1 part extra virgin olive oil in a handy soap dispenser.

Why You'll Like It: It works double duty. Not only do you clean your hands well each time you wash them, but you get a soothing, all-natural moisturizer, too.

17 HANG UP HOT FLASHES Menopausal woes can and do often include pesky hot flashes or temperature ups and downs before, during, and after menopause, aka "The Change." In Asian countries, hot flashes are not a frequent problem according to research because women consume soy, which may help keep hot flashes at bay.

What Oil Remedy to Use: Take 1 or 2 tablespoons of olive oil per day. Or, drizzle a tablespoon or 2 on five servings of vegetables daily. (Include asparagus, beans, carrots, corn, dried seaweed, garlic, green pepper, onions, squash, and yams.)

Why You'll Like It: By using olive oil with vegetables, you may find yourself at a normal temperature rather than feeling waves of heat or turning red while onlookers stare at you as though you were an alien from another planet.

18 LACKLUSTER LIBIDO Not in the mood? You may have read that olive oil can rev up your sex drive or jump-start your (or your lover's) libido. I haven't found any data to prove that olive oil is the cure-all for a lackluster love life, but I do know there are studies that showed sexual performance was enhanced after taking a variety of nutrients including vitamins A, C, E, and B complex and the minerals selenium and zinc. And remember, olive oil is rich in vitamin E (an antioxidant believed to be a sex vitamin).

What Oil Remedy to Use: Eat a low-fat, nutrient-rich meal and drizzle olive oil over it on a regular basis and before a lovemaking session. Also, some people believe porcini olive oil (fresh wild mushrooms infused in olive oil) may act as an aphrodisiac.

Why You'll Like It: Pairing olive oil with a nutrient-dense diet (or porcini olive oil) may do the trick in the bedroom. A healthful, low-fat diet may help to maintain your blood vessels and blood flow, claim medical doctors. That's important in enhancing healthful orgasms in both men and women.

19 MASSAGE MUSCLE ACHES Ever suffer from a strained muscle due to working out at the gym or doing too much indoor or outdoor housework? Actually, muscle aches and pains can affect you at any age. After swimming laps at a resort pool, bringing in plenty of hardwood for a winter fire, walking the dogs, and vacuuming (whew!), my upper back and inner shoulders throbbed. I called a local personal trainer, and he suggested calling a masseuse. Her fee: $120 per hour. I decided to try a healing oil and my own two hands.

What Oil Remedy to Use: Warm 1 cup of olive oil in the microwave. Apply it as a massage oil. (If you have a significant other, this can be even more delightful. But doing it solo can work, too.)

Why You'll Like It: The warmth of the oil immediately relaxes stiff muscles, and the massage motion also loosens up tight muscles and tendons. Plus, you can spend that hundred bucks in multiple other ways to pamper yourself, such as to join a gym that has a hot tub, steam room, and sauna—other ways to soothe your aches and pains away.

The Magic of Scents, Massage, and Oil

Did you know that using olive oil combined with essential oils from aromatic plants can help you to relax the body, mind, and spirit? This isn't news. The art of using aromatic essential oils for physical and mental well-being goes back to the Egyptians. Some of the popular oils for good health include chamomile, lavender, lemon, jasmine, peppermint, rosemary, tea tree, and sandalwood.

To use essential oils, like these powerful healers, you'll need to use a "carrier oil," that is, any oil that is used to dilute pure essential oils. Carrier oils help essential oils spread more evenly, and they help conserve the use of costly essential oils. A common dilution is 10 to 15 drops of essential oil to 1 ounce of carrier oil. Carrier oils are extracted from nuts, kernels, seeds, and other parts of plants.

Almond oil and sesame oil are used for massage. Olive oil is used for healing and lubricating the skin, as well as for massage.

According to massage therapists, there are different types of massage. Here are the most common types:

- Stroking—uses long and firm strokes using the hands or thumbs to trace the outer shape of the body.
- Kneading—works on different muscle groups by lifting, rolling, and squeezing them.
- Friction—uses circular strokes on the deeper muscles and tendons. This technique moves against the grain of a muscle.
- Percussion—uses gentle drumming motions, often on the back.
- Vibration—shakes the muscles back and forth.

Callie's Reviving Massage Oil

This activating eucalyptus massage oil is effective for sore and aching muscles. Combine the following essential oils:

20 drops eucalyptus
20 drops lavender
20 drops rosewood
5 drops chamomile
5 drops peppermint

Add 36 drops of this blend to 3 ounces olive oil. Shake briefly, and massage a small amount into tired, achy muscles and joints.

20 LOSE LICE It seems like kids pick up these pesky creatures at school. The question is, can olive oil be a lice buster or not? Frankly, the answer is not conclusive. Olive oil can zap lice sometimes, sometimes not. So, the verdict is out whether the olive oil remedy is 100 percent effective.

What Oil Remedy to Use: Apply olive oil to the hair and leave it on at least a half hour, according to folks who claim this home cure can do the job. Then, shampoo twice. You may have to try a series of olive oil applications to the head. Olive oil applicator bottles can be purchased at www.headliceinfo.com, where you can also find out everything else you ever wanted to know about lice but were afraid to ask.

Why You'll Like It: If this natural suffocating agent does work for you or your child, you'll be happy because olive oil is a much gentler treatment than the harsh commercial products, which contain pesticides.

21 PEEL AWAY PSORIASIS Psoriasis (which can be worse than lice, which is a short-term problem) can range from mild, in which a few small red patches appear on the elbows or feet, to severe, with unsightly, scaly areas covering the entire body. A friend of mine told me that her cousin suffered from psoriasis, and it truly is more than a cosmetic problem for some people, according to the National Psoriasis Foundation.

What Oil Remedy to Use: Before bedtime, apply olive oil generously to the affected area, then massage. Rinse in the morning. Repeat as needed.

Why You'll Like It: One mom, Jackie Larson of Dallas, Texas, attests that olive oil did the trick. "My son had terrible inherited psoriasis in his scalp. A hairdresser saw this and suggested rubbing olive oil deeply into his scalp. I applied it liberally to his scalp, enough to get his hair wet with it, completely removing any dried skin and thoroughly massaging it in," she recalls. Jackie left the oil in overnight and washed it out in the morning. "Within a matter of days, the flaking had stopped and within a few weeks, his scalp was essentially clear. We repeat when necessary," she notes.

Also, steroid creams can cause additional thinning of the skin. Olive oil is believed to feel better to apply than petroleum jelly or if it works and you nip psoriasis in the bud you won't have to turn to prescription drugs.

22 SOOTHE A STOMACHACHE Upset tummy? Diarrhea? Some folk remedy fans believe olive oil can put your queasy feelings to rest. Also, Edgar Cayce believed the oil adds to the "elasticity of the functioning of the intestinal tract." It doesn't take a crystal ball for you to sense that the smooth liquid can relax an irritated stomach.

What Oil Remedy to Use: Take 1/4 teaspoon every four hours.

Why You'll Like It: If you are nowhere near a pharmacy or a doctor but you are feeling queasy, you'll love this olive oil cure.

23 STOP SUNBURN Skin woes, whether psoriasis or sunburn, can be a problem that lingers for years. Exposure to the ultraviolet rays of sunlight is the main cause of sunburn. I can personally attest that it can be worse if you live in a high altitude, near water, or in an exotic region such as Hawaii or Mexico. I am fair-skinned and I got bad sunburns (second degree) both in Las Vegas and on the Big Island. Since I certainly don't want to get premature wrinkles or skin cancer, I did wear sunscreen. But sometimes it's just not enough.

What Oil Remedy to Use: According to Firenze, use olive oil to soothe the reddened skin and even the blisters that follow sun exposure.

Why You'll Like It: Well, it won't burn like vinegar does. Plus, the silky texture of olive oil pampers a painful burn without pain or a pesky odor.

24 TEND TENDONITIS Shoulder ache? You may have entered painful tendonitis land when your tendons—which connect muscle to bone—become inflamed the way gum tissue often does. I personally can attest to this painful woe, which affected my shoulders after overdoing it with hand weights. Often, it is exercise-related, especially if you do too much. Research shows that olive oil may lessen the aches and pains of bursitis, in which joints become irritated. Both pains are caused by overuse, often from exercise or tasks that require repetitive motions.

What Oil Remedy to Use: Try 1 tablespoon of olive oil before breakfast. If you want to heal faster, try massaging oil into the tender spots as well.

Why You'll Like It: If it works, you will like the fact that you don't have aches and pains from the inflamed regions. Also, it is easier and less time-consuming than icing, which can work in conjunction with this home remedy.

25 TAME TOENAIL FUNGUS Brittle toenails? Since my mid-thirties, I have had dry and brittle toenails. At one time, I was getting professional pedicures twice a month. The pedicurist, from Vietnam, applied an oil on my toes and fingernails before she applied the polish.

I assumed it was something pricey she had purchased at a wholesale store. When I asked her about the miracle worker (it made my nails smooth and not brittle-appearing), she giggled and pointed to a container of a common grocery store brand of vegetable oil.

What Oil Remedy to Use: Apply olive oil or canola oil (any type of lubricating oil can be beneficial) around your toes and nails. However, pure extra virgin olive oil is believed to enhance skin and nail health.

Why You'll Like It: Olive oil is all natural, and it provides an immediate cosmetic effect. Also, the prescription drug that is advertised on television doesn't have a high success rate, and the fact that it necessitates regular blood tests to test for liver problems seems like a red flag to me. Like me, you may prefer to use the accessible oil, which does appear to help camouflage dry and brittle nails (perhaps it's the antioxidant vitamin E that does this) and an earthy-colored polish (some brands include nail strengthener) rather than tamper with my vital organs.

26 TREAT THAT TOOTHACHE Tooth hurt? If one of your teeth—whether a back molar with a filling or a front capped tooth—is throbbing, the pain isn't fun. You may get images of actor Dustin Hoffman in the 1970s film *Marathon Man* and be willing to turn to a popular old remedy—oil of cloves—until you can get to a dentist who wants to help you.

What Oil Remedy to Use: If you don't have oil of cloves on hand, no worry. Blend 2 tablespoons of whole cloves in a blender until a powder forms. Mix with 1 tablespoon of olive oil. Dab on the tooth as needed.

Why You'll Like It: Oil of cloves is a well-known remedy for toothaches. It can provide temporary relief.

27 SO LONG SAD Ever hear of seasonal affective disorder (SAD), or the "winter blues"? Shorter days, longer nights, and a cold climate, especially without sunshine, can make you feel depressed, lack energy, and pack on the pounds. No, I'm not going to say olive oil is the cure-all for SAD, but I do believe it can help you become energized again if you team it with other remedies.

What Oil Remedy to Use: Each day, for lunch or dinner or both meals, drizzle olive oil on a dark, leafy green salad with plenty of fresh vegetables. To sleep like a baby, take 1 tablespoon of flaxseed before bedtime.

Why You'll Like It: If you eat lots of veggies teamed with olive oil, which can fill you up, you may not fill out. Also, if you get a good night's sleep, you will be less likely to overeat when you're energy fizzles throughout the day. Better sleep will make you feel better, and you're more apt to want to exercise, which can help burn calories and fight winter weight gain and depression.

28 STOP SKIN DAMAGE Toenails often are exposed only in the summertime, but your face is seen daily. During your forties (and earlier if you are fair-skinned), your oil glands become less active, which means moisturizing becomes more important. Although all of the antioxidant skin nutrients are key to younger-looking skin, vitamins A, C, and E—well-touted skin rejuvenators—may play even bigger roles, according to dermatologists and researchers in Melbourne, Australia.

Used topically, olive oil—rich in vitamin E—has benefits such as protecting skin against ultraviolet light and reducing the appearance of fine lines and wrinkles. Used internally, it may even help stall the aging process. Eating foods that contain monounsaturated fats, like olive oil, may prevent skin cell damage. Take a look at ageless beauties like Sophia Loren and Loni Anderson, who have given kudos to olive oil.

What Oil Remedy to Use: Dab olive oil on the areas of the skin and face where wrinkles show, and lightly massage at bedtime. Also, include olive oil, along with other antioxidant-rich foods such as vegetables, fresh fruits, and legumes in your daily menus.

Why You'll Like It: It may work to minimize those laugh lines. Plus, Botox and collagen injections are not cheap and not painless.

29 UNIVERSAL EMERGENCY During Mother Nature's wrath, from tornadoes and hurricanes to snowstorms and earthquakes, it's good to have a cure-all product on hand in case of a power outage. Prepare now by putting together a box of emergency supplies. Make sure to include medications that you, your family, and your pet take, as well as a first-aid kit and handbook.

What Oil Remedy to Use: Purchase a large can of extra virgin olive oil (or two), and store it with your emergency supplies. (Note: Bottles can break during a disaster; plastic can react with oil in time.)

Why You'll Like It: Olive oil has healing powers. Rather than trying to put every type of ailment remedy in your emergency supplies box, it's more practical and cost-effective to have one cure that works for many ailments such as burns, cuts, earaches, and sore muscles.

30 VANQUISH VAGINAL DRYNESS A lackluster sex life for women can be connected to lack of lubrication, which can make lovemaking uncomfortable. Olive oil has been used as a sexual lubricant since historical times, but times change. In the twenty-first century, if you're a woman (or man), you know that lovemaking can sizzle if a woman suffers from vaginal dryness, which can occur because of out-of-whack hormones, not being in the mood, infection, and other physical and psychological reasons. But if you think olive oil is the perfect natural oil-based lubricant, think again.

There are some very important guidelines to consider. For one, oils can damage latex condoms and sex toys. Also, olive oil can often be a woman's worst enemy if she is prone to pesky vaginal infections. Since oil clings, it may be a bacteria magnet.

What Oil Remedy to Use: Olive oil works best as a pre-sex enhancer. That means, use edible oils for a sensual massage, hugging, and cuddling. In addition, olive oil–based foods can be erotic shared in bed. Use olive oil as a sexual lubricant *only* with polyurethane female and male condoms, according to Birth Control–Planned Parenthood of Golden Gate. For self-pleasuring, some men have no complaints about olive oil doing the job.

Why You'll Like It: Use caution when applying olive oil directly to your or your mate's private parts. Before you flaunt olive oil behind closed doors, consult your physician. If you get a thumbs-up, enjoy an all-natural sexual enhancer—both sensual and scentless.

THE GOLDEN SECRETS TO REMEMBER

If it doesn't specify which type of oil to use, go ahead and use your own preference: extra virgin olive oil, virgin olive oil, or canola oil.

Ailment	Oil	What It May Do
Bladder infection	Olive oil	Soothes burning
Bruise	Olive oil	Minimizes damage
Chapped skin	Olive oil	Heals
Constipation	Olive oil	Aids in regularity
Cough	Olive oil	Soothes tickle
Cuticles, dry	Olive oil	Heals torn skin
Dandruff	Olive oil	Fights flakes
Diaper rash	Olive oil	Soothes itching and pain
Earache	Olive oil	Wards off infection and pain
Fibromyalgia	Olive oil and essential oils	Helps reduce aches and pains
Gallbladder stones	Olive oil	Soothes stomach pain
Gingivitis	Olive oil	Reduces swelling and throbbing
Hair loss	Olive oil	Aids in healthier hair and scalp
Hangover	Olive oil	Lessens headache
Hot flashes	Olive oil	Maintains normal temperature

Ailment	Oil	What It May Do
Libido, lackluster	Olive oil	Revs up sex drive
Lice	Olive oil	May smother lice
Muscle aches	Olive oil	Soothes pain
Psoriasis	Olive oil	Gets rid of redness and scaly patches
SAD	Olive oil	Boosts energy
Skin burn	Olive oil	Reduces pain
Stomachache	Olive oil	Soothes intestinal tract
Sunburn	Olive oil	Relieves pain
Tendonitis	Olive oil	Relaxes muscles
Toenail fungus	Olive oil	Smoothes brittle nails
Toothache	Olive oil	Provides temporary pain relief
Universal emergency	Olive oil	Acts as cure-all
Vaginal dryness	Olive oil	Provides lubrication

PART 6

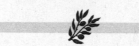

FUTURE OLIVE OIL

Olive Oil Mania: Using Olive Oil for the Household, Kids, Pets, and Beauty

Honor to a Spaniard, no matter how dishonest, is
as real a thing as water, wine, or olive oil.
—Ernest Hemingway[1]

Whether olive oil is used for home cures or heart health, this powerful golden liquid is a household name in the twenty-first century. Not only can you find olive oil in the supermarket (from commercial brands to specialty types), online, and at olive oil tree mills and estates, a variety of olive oil types is cropping up in America and worldwide.

Also, while doctors use it, nutritionists tout it, and plenty of people, like you and me, love its versatility, even conventional associations such as the American Dietetic Association and American Heart Association are giving the "liquid gold" its due kudos.

OLIVE OIL STATISTICS

MAIN OLIVE OIL PRODUCING COUNTRIES IN 2005

Percent of World Supply Produced	Country
36 percent	Spain
25 percent	Italy
18 percent	Greece
8 percent	Tunisia
5 percent	Turkey
4 percent	Syria
3 percent	Morocco
1 percent	Portugal

Source: United Nations Conference on Trade and Development (UNCTAD), www.unctad.org/infocom.

Although olive oil is produced mostly in the Mediterranean countries, it is consumed in Europe, America, and other countries, too, for many reasons—including the heating of the planet.

In *The Sky is Falling! A Global Warming Survival Guide* (AuthorHouse, 2006), my co-author, Mark Jabo, and I wrote: "The coming climatic cataclysm is the new boogeyman on the block and is so serious it's going to get you, your children, and your children's children. It will also affect your second cousin, your cousin's cousin, your children's second cousins, your children's second cousins from a previous marriage, your hamster's hamster, and the clone of your hamster's clone. Whew. Did we leave anyone out?"

Yes, we did forget the sacred olive tree. According to scientists, global warming may affect British olives. Thanks to the heating of the planet (whether humans or nature is to blame), the nation's first olive grove of more than 100 olive trees has been planted in Devon, England, and may begin producing olive oil like in the Mediterranean basin within several years. So, in the future, England may be consuming more of the golden stuff.

MAIN OLIVE OIL CONSUMING COUNTRIES IN 2005

Percent of World Supply Consumed	Country
30 percent	Italy
20 percent	Spain
11 percent	Other non-European
9 percent	Greece
8 percent	United States
5 percent	Other European
3 percent	Syria
2 percent	Algeria
2 percent	Morocco
2 percent	Portugal
2 percent	Tunisia

Source: United Nations Conference on Trade and Development (UNCTAD), www.unctad.org/infocom.

HEALING YOUR HOME ROOM BY ROOM

While olive oil is consumed worldwide, it's also used for a variety of household chores. When I was a teenager, I always cleaned house for my mom, who was one of those working mothers. I remember we had a cleaning lady come into our home twice a month to do the heavy chores such as cleaning the shower and oven. She would use strong chemicals to clean the showers and oven.

That was back in the 1960s. Today, women and men, like you and me, prefer to use more natural stuff rather than subject our bodies, families, pets, and friends to lingering chemicals that have potential side effects.

Are Your Household Cleaners Making You Ill?

Chemical sensitivities—are they real? You bet. These toxic chemicals can and do wreak havoc on people who use them, as well as on people who are in the environment after they are used. If you can use natural cleaners, such as olive oil and vinegar, by all means do so, to avoid these ill effects. Here are seven toxic chemicals that are guaranteed to make you plug your nose or worse.

Cleaning Chemical	Found In	Potential Side Effects
Ammonia	Glass cleaners, floor cleaners, furniture polishes	Irritates the eyes, nose, lungs; causes rashes, redness
Bleach	Disinfectants, laundry bleaches, toilet bowl cleaner	Irritates the skin; when mixed with ammonia, forms a toxic gas
Formaldehyde	Disinfectants, furniture polishes, detergents	Nasal stuffinesss, itchy red eyes, nausea, headache
Glycols	Degreasers, dry cleaning chemicals, floor cleaners	Irritates the skin, eyes, nose, throat
Lye	Tub and tile cleaners	When mixed with acids, can cause harmful vapors; splashed in eyes, can cause blindness
Napthalene	Air fresheners, carpet cleaners	Dangerous to breathe; can cause headaches, nausea, confusion
Petroleum distillates	Air fresheners, carpet cleaners	Dangerous to breathe; can cause headaches, nausea, confusion

Source: The Healing Powers of Vinegar.

Here are some things you can do with olive oil and vinegar teamed with other natural ingredients such as lemon, water, and essential oils. You'll find that these mixtures can be used to clean floors, polish furniture, freshen the air, and much, much more.

Yard

- **Repel Moles.** One individual who calls herself Mrs. FIXIT and provides home repair and household tips claims olive oil can be used to keep moles away. Soak a rag with olive oil and stuff it into the mole hole. I have to battle raccoons every year. Perhaps, a strong-flavored olive oil can do the trick. It's worth a try. (*Source:* Mrs. FIXIT's How-To Library, www.mrsfixit.com.)
- **Prevent Rust.** Mrs. FIXIT also recommends keeping olive oil in the garage as well as inside the home. According to the creative olive oil user, a "quick coat on gardening tools will keep them from rusting. It will also lubricate garage door tracks." Note to self: Use olive oil on snow shovels and rakes.

Living Room

- **Polish Plants.** Houseplants get dull and dusty. Try spraying with a solution of water and olive oil. Not only will you have dust-free leaves, but they will shine. Plus, if you live in a cold, dry climate and mist your plants, it is as good as talking to them.
- **Dust It Dust-Free.** Don't like to dust? Try the Vinegar Institute's all-natural remedy. Mix olive oil and vinegar in a 1-to-1 ratio and polish with a soft cloth. I tried it on my entertainment center (another hand-me-down from my dad), and it is without dust, shines, and doesn't have a chemical odor.
- **Wipe Out Table Rings.** Got rings around your tables? I have a 30-year-old wooden living room table that I adore for sentimental reasons. I noticed a teacup ring on the lower shelf. I mixed a paste of olive oil (extra virgin) and lemon juice (2 parts olive oil to 1 part lemon juice) and applied it to the area using a circular motion, let it sit briefly, and wiped it off. The ring around my table is now gone.
- **Sparkle Up Blinds.** If you want your veneer blinds to shine like

they did when you first put them up, I recommend olive oil. After you dust them, wipe them with a wet cloth dipped in gentle, soapy water, rinse, and dry. Then, apply a light coat of olive oil, and polish for a brief time, until they look like new again.

• **Love Leather Furniture.** I hesitated to use olive oil on my new, pricey leather sofa, love seat, and oversized chair. But I also didn't want to purchase a product containing harsh chemicals. The Vinegar Institute recommends a solution of distilled white vinegar and linseed oil. (I recommend olive oil.) Gently rub this protector onto your favorite leather items and rub gently with a cloth.

• **Clean Candleholders**. Do you have melted wax built up on your candleholders? No problem. Mix a solution of olive oil and mild dish soap. It takes off old wax and grime, and leaves brass, ceramic, and colored metal candleholders shining brightly.

• **Lighten Up with Lamps.** In ancient times, olive oil was used as fuel for olive oil lamps. Today, you still can purchase oil lamps—all kinds—and use them in the living room. Cabin lamps are bright and radiate more light than other lamps, such as a chamber lamp (which can be taken from room to room) or a table lamp (used for ambiance to see your clean home).

Olive Oil Keeps on Burning

So, why in the world would you use an olive oil lamp in this day and age? For starters, "They are safer than candles, because the flame is enclosed. They are also more efficient and provide better light because they don't flicker as much as candles. And they don't create any smoke or odor, for those using non-electric lighting in an enclosed area if you have allergies," explains Glenda Lehman Ervin, daughter of the founder of Lehman's Lamps. But that's not all . . .

There are a variety of perks to burning olive oil in the twenty-first century. Here are five reasons why olive oil makes a great fuel, according to the booklet *I Didn't Know That Olive Oil Would Burn!* by Merry Bickers:

1. Vegetarians and animal rights folks can sleep at night knowing that olive oil is a natural, animal-free product.

2. Religious people enjoy olive oil for its traditional use.
3. Olive oil is fume-free and a much better option for people who are sensitive to the fumes from petroleum fuels.
4. If you're on a budget, olive oil is a cost-effective fuel. For lamp fuel, you can use any kind of olive oil or can buy it in bulk, which can cut the cost.
5. Olive oil as a lamp fuel is much safer than petroleum-based fuels, which can ignite into a flame. (But note, all flames can be dangerous, and none should be left unattended, especially around young children or pets.)

Dining Room

- **Buff Brass.** To keep brass looking shinier, buff knickknacks with olive oil after cleaning them. I have a hand-me-down collection from my dad, who was also a nature lover. So, preserving his brass birds and reindeer means a lot to me. Olive oil keeps the brass from tarnishing so fast.
- **Preserve Antiques.** I have a glass dining room table with classic wrought iron from the good old 1950s. Rubbing a bit of extra virgin olive oil onto the iron legs of the table and four chairs using a soft cloth provides a fantastic shine to this classic and preserves its worth.

Kitchen

- **Cutting Board Cleanup.** A wooden cutting board in your kitchen is a must-have, and olive oil can help to preserve it. After using it, wash it in soap and water. Dry. Then, once it is squeaky clean, wipe it with olive oil.
- **No More Rust.** Got a cast-iron frying pan? If so, chances are it's a hand-me-down. So, you want to take care of it and keep it in tip-top condition. After each time you use it, wash it, and dry it, don't forget to lightly apply olive oil to keep it rust-free and maintain its natural shine.
- **Pamper Kitchen Helpers.** Olive oil fans use the versatile home aid to add a vibrant shine to kitchen helpers such as the blender, coffeemaker, and stainless steel toaster. After you clean these items, simply spray them with a mist of olive oil and water (3 parts water to 1 part olive oil) and buff until they gleam olive oil pretty.

Bedroom

- **Dust Delights.** Wooden furniture in your bedroom? You certainly don't want to smell chemicals from furniture polish with toxins, right? If you want to keep your personal sanctuary dust-free and smelling fragrant, use a mixture of olive oil and fresh lemon juice for the bed, nightstands, framed mirror, and picture frames.

Bathroom

- **Remove Dirt on Bathroom Floors.** Got a natural bathroom floor that could use a nice shine without the buildup of wax? After I washed my low-maintenance, all-natural-looking, neutral-colored slate floor, I mixed a few drops of olive oil with fresh lemon juice and wiped the floor once again. Ah, the fragrance and shine were enough to make me vow to never use a floor wax.
- **Polish Pretty Bathroom Treasures.** To add a nice, lasting shine to the ceramic figurines often found in a bathroom, use 3 parts olive oil and 1 part water. Buff until your treasures look bright and clean.

Family Room

- **Wow Wood-Paneling Scratches.** I live in a house that was built in 1931. It has a lot of built-in cupboards, and it's wood paneled throughout, including in the family room. I use a traditional furniture polish first and then buff surface scratches with olive oil. This makes the paneling appear scratch-free.
- **Freshen Wood.** Speaking of wood paneling, I love it. To keep it looking its best, mix 1 ounce of olive oil with 2 ounces of white vinegar and 1 quart of warm water. Dampen a soft cloth with the solution and wipe the paneling. Then, wipe with a dry, soft cloth to remove yellowing from the surface.

Home Office

- **Get a Grime Fighter.** Black picture frames in your home office? As I looked at William Shakespeare and Einstein as well as my Barnes & Noble events posters, I decided to buff the frames with olive oil. They shine and look clean.

Laundry Room

- **Good-bye to Scratchy Lingerie.** If you have cotton underpants, I recommend mixing a solution of olive oil and mild detergent. Then handwash. Say bye-bye to expensive commercial fabric softeners, which often have strange, unnatural scents.

HEALTHY KID STUFF

When I think about children, Gemma Sanita Sciabica comes to mind. On the telephone, we discussed the topic of parents cooking healthy and how that will help their children to grow up healthy. Gemma sent me a card in which she wrote: "It is a good idea to watch children's diet making sure they do not have too much cholesterol. Using olive oil more, will prevent problems later."

- **It's Time for Pizza.** So, I thought, "Kids love pizza." Rather than order a pizza from a fast-food chain, why not make it a family night and create a healthy and tasty pie with olive oil and plenty of healthy toppings so both girls and boys can bake and choose. Here is one of Gemma's delightful pizza recipes.

Pizza Dough

1¼ cups water (110°)
1 package dry yeast
3½–4 cups flour

¾ teaspoon salt
¼ cup Marsala Olive Fruit Oil
1 egg white

In mixing bowl, add ¼ cup water and dry yeast. Let stay about 10 minutes. In another bowl, add dry ingredients. Make well in center and pour in yeast mixture, oil, remaining water, and egg white. Stir to mix into a smooth, pliable dough. On lightly floured board, knead for several minutes. Place dough back in lightly oiled bowl, cover, and put in a warm place for about 1 hour or until doubled. Turn dough out on floured board and cut into desired sizes.

Place toppings of your choice on top of dough, then leave to rise about 20 minutes or until dough is puffy. Drizzle with olive oil. Bake in 375° oven for 20–30 minutes or until crust is golden. Makes one 15-x-10-inch or two 12-inch pies.

Variation: Substitute 1 cup whole wheat, semolina, or cornmeal flour for white flour. Add ¼ cup wheat germ.

Topping Combinations

- Fresh tomatoes, fresh garlic, grilled vegetables, fresh herbs, and feta or Gorgonzola cheese
- Pesto (brushed on crust), provolone, ricotta cheese, Romano cheese, fresh tomatoes, roasted garlic, and grilled mushrooms
- Grilled lemon herb chicken, roasted potatoes, and dried ricotta cheese or provolone
- Fresh tomatoes, fresh or canned clams, garlic, parsley, basil, oregano, black and red hot pepper flakes, and Romano cheese

(*Source: Cooking with California Olive Oil: Treasured Family Recipes* by Gemma Sanita Sciabica)

- **It's Time for Pasta.** *Lunch Lessons'* author Ann Cooper, former executive chef of the Putney Inn in Vermont and former president and current board member of Women's Chefs and Restauranteurs, says: "Orzo is a nice little pasta that is great in salads and side dishes. We love the fresh flavors of the herbs and lemon juice. Enlist your children to help you experiment with different herbs and vegetables by asking them to come up with some of their favorite combinations. Send this to school as a side dish to a wrap sandwich. If you want to enhance the nutritional value of this salad use whole wheat orzo."

Orzo Salad

❖ ❖ ❖

1 pound orzo-pasta
5 tablespoons chopped fresh
  oregano
5 tablespoons chopped fresh mint
  leaves

6 tablespoons olive oil
3 tablespoons fresh lemon juice
½ teaspoon salt
Fresh ground black pepper as
  needed

Cook orzo in boiling water until tender, drain, and put in a large mixing bowl. Add oregano and mint, and toss to combine. In a small bowl, combine the oil and lemon juice, and add to orzo mixture, mixing well. Season with salt and pepper. Serves 8.

Nutrition Facts
Serving Size 1 serving
Servings Per Recipe 8
Amount Per Serving

	%Daily Value
Calories 175	
Calories from fat 97 (55% of total cal)	
Total fat 11 g	17%
Saturated fat 2 g	8%
Cholesterol 23 mg	8%
Sodium 196 mg	8%
Total Carbohydrate 18 mg	6%
Dietary Fiber 2 g	6%
Sugars 16 g	
Protein 3 g	
Vitamin A 39%	**Vitamin C 10%**
Calcium 7%	Iron 25%

*Percent Daily Values are based on a 2,000 calorie diet. Your daily values may be higher or lower depending upon your caloric intake.

- **It's Time for Pie.** Fun for kids doesn't have to stop in the kitchen. Do you remember playing outdoors as a child and being able to pick fresh berries, apples, or apricots from trees in an orchard or in your own backyard? While the twenty-first century might be keeping children busy at the computer, why not join them in a nature walk and gather fresh berries? Gemma told me no-roll pie crusts are not as time-consuming to make as traditional rolled pie crusts, the type my mom used to make. (However, if you want to try a double crust or whole wheat crust, get a copy of Gemma's *Baking Sensational Sweets with California Olive Oil*.) So, here is a non-traditional olive oil pie crust recipe that can be used for tart shells and fresh berry pies (recipe follows). Let the good times roll.

No-Roll Pie Crust
9-10 or 11 inch

❖ ❖ ❖

1½ *cups flour*
2 *tablespoons sugar*
1 *teaspoon baking powder*

½ *teaspoon salt*
¼ *cup milk*
½ *cup Marsala Olive Oil*

Preheat oven to 375°. In mixing bowl, add dry ingredients and make well in center. Pour in milk and add olive oil. Stir with fork until just combined. Gather into a ball, flatten slightly, and place in bottom of 9-inch tart pan with removable bottom.

With floured fingertips, press from center out to edge. Using the bottom of a floured ¼- cup measuring cup, press dough firmly against sides of pan. Form an edge with thumb and finger, making a small rim. Pierce bottom with fork to prevent puffing during baking. Bake 15–17 minutes or until golden. Cover edge with pie crust rim or foil if browning too quickly.

Note: For a thinner 9-inch crust, remove ¼ cup dough before pressing dough into pie pan. For a 10- or 11-inch pie crust, use dough as is. I tried to change the amounts of the ingredients in this crust, but it didn't come out as good. Now I make the crust using the amounts stated and remove the ¼ cup of dough for the 9-inch crust. No one will mind your bending from tradition when you make this no-roll pie crust. It is simple, tasty, and flaky. We really like it a lot.

To make 4-inch tart shells, press about 3 tablespoons of dough into each tart pan. Bake about 10 minutes or until golden. Fill with your favorite filling fruits. (See Fresh Berry Pie below.)

(*Source:* by Gemma Sanita Sciabica, *Baking Sensational Sweets with California Olive Oil*)

Fresh Berry Pie

1 cup sugar
3 tablespoons cornstarch or tapioca flour
4 cups boysenberries (or berries of your choice)

¼ teaspoon cinnamon
2 tablespoons lemon juice
1 olive oil pie crust dough (double)

Mix sugar and cornstarch, and toss with berries, cinnamon, and lemon juice. Turn into pastry lined pie plate. Bake in a 425° oven 35–45 minutes or until golden brown. Makes 9-inch pie.

(*Source:* by Gemma Sanita Sciabica, *Baking Sensational Sweets with California Olive Oil*)

Pets and Olive Oil

1 **Smooth a Pooch's Snout** Olive oil can help soothe chapped human lips, so why not use it to soothe a canine nose cracked from chilly weather? As a Lake Tahoe resident who knows what cold, dry air does to my skin, I can tell you that oil may be helpful to dogs' cold noses. My two Brittanys love the snow. If their paws can become dry and cracked from the cold, dry ground, why not their tender black noses?

   What Oil Remedy to Use: Use a small amount of extra virgin olive oil (only the best for our pets, right?) on your dog's nose and gently massage it.

   Why You'll Like It: You'll see a smooth, shiny surface. The best part is, it's natural and doesn't have a scent.

2 Fight Ticks Back in the good old days, when I hitchhiked across America with my black Labrador retriever Stonefox (it was a common phenomenon in the 1970s), I recall that in mountain regions, a tick or two sometimes would find their way into his coat. Looking at the rounded body of the tick would make me squirm, while my dog didn't know the difference. I'd light a match to it and pray that the tick would work its way out of my canine's fur as I lightly pulled on it. But there are better remedies.

What Oil Remedy to Use: It's less dangerous using gentle olive oil than holding a lighted match to your best friend. Plus, as *The Passionate Olive* author Carol Firenze notes, "Ticks breathe oxygen, and they can be suffocated with a coat of olive oil."[2]

Why You'll Like It: In the film *City of Angels*, Maggie (Meg Ryan), a surgeon, must remove a tick from her yellow Lab. Her doctor-boyfriend's first recommendation is alcohol. When Maggie claims she doesn't have any hospital stuff in her home, he inquires about olive oil. She offers jalapeño or rosemary. It was a dab of rosemary olive oil that was the oil of choice and did the trick to remove the tick.

3 Ice Balls Last winter, my brother would take Simon, my fun-loving pooch, for long walks in the deep, snowy field and campground. He'd bring back my long-coated orange-and-white Brittany all wet, with his foot pads and stomach sporting ice balls that would matt his fur. Into the warm shower we'd go. Isn't there an easier solution?

What Oil Remedy to Use: Firenze seems to think so. She says to fill a plastic spray bottle with olive oil and "spritz it on the fur" to zap the ice and snow and smooth the fur. My first reaction was "No way!" I've witnessed these thick ice balls, and warm water does the trick. However, spraying olive oil on a dog's coat afterwards is a good idea, since it keeps the fur soft and conditioned.[3]

Why You'll Like It: Naturally, it would be a godsend if Firenze's remedy worked. Note to self: Spray extra virgin olive oil (nothing but the best for my two boys) on their coats next snow day. However, I will have fresh towels ready for warm-water applications or a shower just in case. P.S.: I will also use that olive oil spritz on my hands, to keep them soft after tending to the dogs.

4 **Gooey Foot Pads** Uh-oh. Did Fluffy or Fido step in something sticky such as gum or tar? This sticky situation can be frustrating for both pet and caretaker. So, what can you do rather than watch your poor cat or dog lick and chew the unwanted substance? Olive oil comes to the rescue.

What Oil Remedy to Use: Try soaking the foot pad in a solution of warm saltwater and olive oil. The two ingredients may break up the foreign substance, and both the oil and the salt may also soothe any redness.

Why You'll Like It: Using a natural salt–olive oil solution may do the trick, especially if the substance doesn't cover the entire foot pad. If it works, it beats cutting the fur, ignoring the situation, or watching your companion animal struggle to make it better while it only gets worse. Plus, a home cure that gets a thumbs-up is preferred to a pricey vet visit.

5 **Clean Ears** Dogs and cats can get ear mites, small parasitic creatures that take up residence in their ears, causing itching and inflammation. Olive oil or a natural product that contains it, whether you use it to prevent a case of ear mites or to treat it, may help ease the itch and fight the infection.

What Oil Remedy to Use: Firenze recommends olive oil because it will "drown the mites." You can dab olive oil on a cotton ball and rub gently inside and outside your pet's ear canal. Or, you can use an olive oil–based natural pet product for ear mites.[4]

Why You'll Like It: Well, it's natural. And if it does work, it is better than ignoring the problem and then having to pay a professional to treat it when it becomes a pesky problem that neither you nor your pet can tune out.

6 **Cancer Fighter** Cats and dogs over 10 years of age (and even younger) can receive the earth-shattering diagnosis of cancer. But as frightened as they may become, I know pet lovers are not powerless. When my 18-year-old cat developed cancer, surgery bought him more time. But pets, like people, can also take advantage of a holistic arsenal—herbs, homeopathy, natural nutrition, and dietary supplements—to prevent and treat cancer.

What Oil Remedy to Use: Add olive oil to your pet's diet. It will help prevent free-radical damage to cells, which can lead to abnormal cell growth. Consult with a holistic veterinarian regarding the amount, since it will vary depending on the weight of the cat or dog.

Why You'll Like It: Using natural cancer fighters like olive oil in your pet's daily diet regimen will help you be proactive.

7 **Canine Chow** A devout olive oil fan who calls herself "The Garden Lady" told me, "Olive oil should be in everyone's dog dish." She insists it makes her dog's coat shiny, "and he thinks he's getting 'people food.' I make a production of taking the bottle off the counter that's next to the stove, so he knows that he's getting some of our provisions. The plain chow he won't eat, but the chow with olive oil is absolutely inhaled."

What Oil Remedy to Use: Put 1 teaspoon of olive oil in your dog's food daily. Note: Consult with your veterinarian first to make sure the amount is appropriate for your pet, since the weight of a 5-pound teacup poodle is different than that of a large Labrador retriever.

Why You'll Like It: If you go to a holistic vet, chances are olive oil will get a thumbs-up. However, a conventional vet may tell you that there is no reason to include the oil in your pet's diet or may suggest a commercial brand of essential fatty acids to add to your dog's food.

8 **Dog and Cat Shampoo** Ever consider adding olive oil to your pet's shampoo? It's not unheard of, at all. The olive oil may keep

the skin healthy and leave the coat shining, according to people who make and/or use the oil in pet grooming products. Also, it may help maintain good skin hydration and even prevent matting on a long-haired canine.

What Oil Remedy to Use: Mix 1/2 teaspoon with your pet's recommended amount of natural shampoo. Massage in, then rinse.

Why You'll Like It: If you're like me, you may prefer to use olive oil topically on your pet rather than to include it in your pet's food. It's a quick, all-natural way to keep your dog's coat looking good and feeling great. Note: I did massage a dab of olive oil into Simon's dry coat (like I did for my own hair) and followed with a brushing. The outcome: His coat appeared a bit on the oily side. The second day, it looked like he was having a good canine hair day.

9 **Use Natural Dog Treats** Want to give your dog (or cat) a special edible treat but don't want chemicals? No problem. In fact, did you know that there are natural products on the market that actually contain olive oil?

What Oil Remedy to Use: Most supermarkets don't have a wide selection of natural pet treats, but if you're lucky (read the labels), you may find one or two brands. I purchased one brand at the grocery store, and it contained canola oil.

Why You'll Like It: If you don't like eating foods with chemicals and preservatives, you probably want to feed your pets all-natural goodies, too. Once you find a brand they like, you'll be pleased to know that it's a good and healthful snack for your animal angels. Or, if you want to be sure your critters get olive oil–based treats, you can make them yourself.

10 **Make Olive Oil Goodies** Wish you had an easy-to-bake dog biscuit recipe? Online, you'll find a variety of homemade pet treats, and in some natural pet-care books, you'll also find recipes that include olive oil.

What Oil Remedy to Use: I suggest using extra virgin olive oil because you want to give the best to your best friend, right? Some recipes call for 2 tablespoons of olive oil.

Why You'll Like It: "We use olive oil because it is such an excellent source of omega fatty acids, and typically, in the diet of today's dog, essential fatty acids (EFAs) are sadly lacking," say the dog experts at www.knowbetterdogfood.com. Plus, vets will tell you that if your dog's coat lacks shine, your companion animal may be lacking EFAs.

Adds the Two Dog Press expert: "We use olive oil in our treat recipes because I use olive oil almost exclusively in my cooking for humans. It's what I always have available in the cupboard. Plus, it's a rich source of good, healthy, vegetable-based fat and it adds more flavor than corn or safflower oils."

Dog Biscuits They'll Roll Over For!

❖ ❖ ❖

LIVER DOG BISCUITS

3 cups oat flour
½ cup pureed fresh liver (beef or chicken) or 1 tablespoon dessicated liver powder
1 egg
2 tablespoons olive oil
Water or chicken or beef broth to moisten

CHEESE DOG BISCUITS

3 cups oat flour
1 cup grated Cheddar cheese
1 egg
2 tablespoons olive oil
Water to moisten

In a large bowl, add all the ingredients. Mix well, form into a ball, and roll out to a ¼-inch thickness with a rolling pin. Cut into desired shapes, place on cookie sheets, and bake in a 325° oven for about 30 minutes or until well browned. Turn off the oven, leaving the biscuits in the oven until cooled.

These biscuits can be frozen, but keep well for a couple of weeks if they are very dry and crisp. Most dog biscuits contain wheat or corn, which can be allergens for dogs. This recipe uses oat flour as an alternative. Do not use raisins in the recipe, as raisins and grapes can be fatal to dogs. Onions and garlic are also toxic. Bon Appétit!

(*Source:* www.knowbetterdogfood.com)

Big Boy Beef Biscuits

❖ ❖ ❖

½ cup dry milk
1 egg
1 teaspoon parsley
6 tablespoons olive oil
2 teaspoons honey

1 small (2.5-ounce) jar beef baby food
½ cup beef broth
1 cup whole wheat flour
½ cup rye flour
½ cup rice flour
½ cup cracked wheat

Glaze
1 egg
2 tablespoons beef broth

Preheat oven to 325°. In a large bowl, combine the dry milk, egg, parsley, oil, honey, baby food, and broth. Gradually blend in the flours and cracked wheat. Add enough wheat flour to form a stiff dough. Transfer to a floured surface and knead until smooth, about 3–5 minutes. Shape the dough into a ball and roll to 1/2-inch thick. Using bone-shaped cookie cutters, make biscuits. Transfer to ungreased baking sheets, spacing about 1/4 inch apart. Gather up the scraps, roll out again, and cut additional biscuits. Bake for 30 minutes. Whisk together the egg and broth for the glaze. Brush biscuits with the glaze on both sides. Return to oven and bake for an additional 30 minutes. Let cool overnight.

Makes several dozen small bones or 2½–3 dozen large bones, depending on the size of the cookie cutter.

(*Source:* Two Dog Press http://www.twodogpress.com/dogfood.html)

Now that we've put popular olive oil on the table and explained how to use it to make a happy home and maintain healthy kids and pets, take a look at how the versatile oil—either by itself or as an ingredient in ready-made beauty products—can help to beautify you from head to toe.

The Golden Secrets to Remember

✓ Spain, Italy, and Greece are the top olive oil producing countries in the world as well as the top consumers.

✓ Olive oil can be used to heal your home in a variety of amazing ways.

✓ If you have chemical sensitivities or care about using eco-friendly cleaning products inside and outside your home, olive oil is the choice for you.

✓ It's never too soon to teach your kids how to eat and cook healthy. Olive oil can help you do just that.

✓ Olive oil is an all-purpose natural remedy for both cats and dogs that can provide better health and edible treats.

Olive Beautiful

*His branches shall spread, and his beauty shall be
as the olive tree.*

—Bible[1]

The only thing better than pampering your home and pets is spoiling
yourself. When I was a kid, my grandmother allowed us to take deep,
lukewarm bubble baths in the middle of hot summer days. She'd bring
in snacks for us to nibble on, from cold cuts, which included fresh carrots, celery, cherry tomatoes, and both black and green olives, and tall
glasses of iced tea.

Today, spa resorts and day spas offer a variety of pampering treats.
But you can get the same benefits right at home. A bathtub (or shower),
quality time, and the right olive oil–based cosmetics and soaps are all
you need.

Olive oil itself and ready-made products come in the form of bath
oil, body gel, hand lotion, lip balm, shampoo, crème rinse, and soap.
Thanks to my research, I've tried each and every one of them. And because I'm a natural woman, I am hooked on the magic of olive oil for
beauty.

For centuries, Mediterranean women have turned to olive oil to
condition their hair, making it shine. Italian actress Sophia Loren, at
71, told the media that the secret to her youthful looks is "the odd
bath in virgin olive oil." Olive oil has been used for skin treatments since

biblical times—and in the twenty-first century, it's finding its way back as a beauty product around the world.

While women and men have countless beauty products to use, I decided to try some ready-made olive oil–based soaps to see if they are worth the "gold" that the oil once was in historical times.

THE OLIVE AND THE BEAUTY

Olive Oil Soaps:
L'Olivier Bar Soap

Elie Maghames, owner of the Sonoma, California–based company L'Olivier, sent me several of his 80 different soaps. As an Ivory girl forever, I was hesitant to try something new. But after sniffing the box containing a bar of lavender soap, I opened it. Pleased with its natural fragrance, I used it in my morning shower. It was a heavenly experience. The scent and silky feel of the soap on my feet, legs, torso, and arms was amazing. I was hooked.

Shampoos and Conditioners:
Baronessa Cali Body Building Shampoo
Baronessa Cali Conditioner

These were part of a gift. I used both. I do have my favorite shampoos (the kind that promise full and thick hair), but I confess these products with "extracts of Italian Olive Oil" left my hair soft (yes, incredibly silky) and nice to touch, while my curly locks are prone to dryness in the winter months and due to the chlorine from swimming in both indoor and outdoor pools year round.

Olive Oil Lotions and Gels:
Baronessa Cali Hand and Body Moisturizer
Baronessa Cali Shower and Bath Gel

As with the olive oil soap, I am in love with my Cali hand and body lotion. The torn cuticles on my hands every winter are nonexistent this time around. In the morning and at night at work in my study, I use it religiously. Plus, I prefer a natural-based hand and body lotion rather than one with ingredients I can't pronounce. So, without doubt, this Cali lotion works for me.

I don't often use gels in the shower, but it is a treat to do so. It's something I will do if I go to a spa or when I travel and pamper myself at a plush hotel. So, to be able to use a product like this, and a natural good-for-you one, is a treat, and like the other Cali products, it made my skin feel smooth, clean, and pampered.

The Man Behind Extra Virgin Olive Oil Soaps

Who in the olive oil world makes and sells only olive oil soaps? Meet Elie Maghames, 50, a charming Lebanon-born man who grew up in France. In America for nearly 20 years, he opened up the olive oil store L'Olivier in Sonoma, California, in 2001. The ambitious entrepreneur sold fifty types of olive oils and vinegars. By 2004, he noticed it was his olive oil soaps that were the moneymakers.

"After tasting all of the olive oil, we didn't like some, and we thought they weren't good enough for our customers, so we started making olive oil soap," points out Maghames. A few months passed, and they provided only ten fragrances, while there were daily requests to add more scents. Nowadays, L'Olivier has about eighty fragrances. Many of these soaps are made with extra virgin olive oil.

Some of the natural essential oil fragrances include: grapefruit, lime, lavender, lavender/clove/orange, lavender/lime, lavender/eucalyptus/tea tree, oatmeal/lavender/peppermint, orange, patchouli, and rosemary/sage.

These days, you can find Maghames selling only soaps and skin care products, such as olive oil soaps, olive massage oils, lip salves, and specialty soaps. In fact, his business is growing, so he will be relocating to a larger, factory-type building to continue his work.

With a French accent and down-to-earth manner, Maghames freely talks about his products and their unique qualities. He believes olive oil is one of the few oils that goes deep into the skin without clogging the pores. It attracts moisture to the skin and prevents it from drying.

"Growing up around the Mediterranean Sea, I was amazed to see ladies of all ages using olive oil on their hair and skin daily. Their hair was fluffy and healthy, and their bodies were very soft. My grandma used to tell me: 'If the oil can protect inside your body, why not the outside,'" recalls Maghames.

This modest olive oil soap maker is hardly alone. He has loyal buyers located on the West Coast and in the Pacific Northwest, the Southern Midwest, and Europe, too. These are quotes from customers who use Maghames' olive oil soap:

I was given a bar of L'Olivier olive oil soap as a gift. It is a lovely product. I tried one bar that was given to me and liked it enough that I ordered several bars online. I have tried using the soap on my face—it gently cleans make-up off and leaves your skin feeling moisturized—but not greasy. I have also used it on my arms and legs with great results. Small skin blemishes on my arms are gone. I love this product, and will order more in the future.
—Ellie McMillan, WA

I'm a guy who would have never purchased anything but Lever 2000 but my girlfriend introduced me to the soap and I've been hooked ever since! I had mild eczema but since using the soap, I have not had any flare-ups at all in the past three years—it's really amazing. My skin is awesome! So much for those $200 creams from the pharmacy.
—Edward M. Marcel, Replenishment Buyer, Longs Drug Stores

Beauty Tips from Head to Toe

Ready-made products are a treat because they're convenient and smell nice. But, using olive oil by itself or with other ingredients from your kitchen cupboards can work wonders, too. In fact, using both olive oil out of a bottle and ready-made olive oil–based soaps and skin care products is like having the best of both worlds. Go ahead—try using olive oil solo for your crowning glory to your tender feet.

- **Soft and Shiny Hair.** Fatty acid–rich olive oil can penetrate the hair cuticle and smooth dry hair. Celebrity hairstylists and beauty experts recommend putting a few drops of olive oil in the palm of your hand and rubbing until the skin glistens. Then, work the oil into your locks, starting at the ends.

I did this months ago—first with canola oil and then with extra virgin olive oil. Both oils do the trick. Your hair, especially if it's exposed to a cold, dry climate, chlorine, blow dryers, curling irons, or hair products, will be softer and silkier to touch, and it will appear less dry and have a nice sheen.

- **Hair Conditioner.** Looking for a deep conditioning treatment for dry hair? Combine 1/4 cup extra virgin olive oil with 1/4 cup spring water. Massage into your dry hair, and cover with a plastic bag. Wait 20 minutes, shampoo, and use your regular hair conditioner.

- **Skin Moisturizer.** Many women have told me that they use extra virgin olive oil on their face at night as a moisturizer. In the morning, I use an all-purpose moisturizing crème with SPF 15. At night, I use the olive oil nighttime remedy. I apply the oil to my face, around my eyes, and on my laugh lines (and the extra I rub into my hands and cuticles). In the morning, my skin feels softer than usual. A bonus: Antiaging crèmes cost $15 and up. This remedy costs less—and may do more.

- **Eye Makeup Remover.** If you wear eyeliner, mascara, and eye shadow, like women do to enhance their eyes, you also know that it is a task to remove these beauty enhancers. An easy-does-it eye makeup remover may be as close to you as your kitchen cabinet. Try mixing 1 tablespoon of canola oil with 1 tablespoon of extra virgin olive oil. Apply a small amount to a cotton ball and wipe your eyelashes and eyelids.

- **Smooth Shaving Cream.** Olive oil fans insist the oil can be used to shave. Not only does it moisturize, but it will soften the hair and make the procedure more comfy for a man's beard or woman's legs. Try mixing 1 tablespoon of extra virgin olive oil, 1/2 cup of warm water, and 1 tablespoon of a gentle liquid soap. For best results, use a clean, sharp razor.

- **Soften Elbows.** In the spring and summertime, it's common to notice rough elbows. But why not take care of this alligator-type skin year-round? Then, whether it's shower time or bedtime, you'll have one less beauty woe.

  Italy's Antonio recommends his grandmother's easy-to-do remedy. Dip your elbows in a bowl of lukewarm olive oil. (Warm it up in the microwave.) Repeat as needed, and your elbows will become smooth before you can say "soft elbows."

- **Stretch Marks.** Both women and men can get those small, depressed streaks in the skin that appear on the tummy, buttocks, thighs, hips, and breasts. While they are most common on the stomach in the later stages of pregnancy when the belly is quickly expanding, they also can be seen on people who gain weight (or build up muscle) and lose body fat or muscle mass rapidly. Plus, if your mom or dad had stretch marks, you may, too, thanks to the genetic factor.

  To minimize those marks on your body, rub olive oil on the area at least twice daily. When celebrity Brooke Burke had to have a bikini-ready body a few months after childbirth for a photo shoot, she turned to oil during her pregnancy, according to Celebrity Parents (www.celebrityparents.com). "I rubbed oil into my hips, belly and breasts every day, twice a day," she says. "You can use shea butter, cocoa butter, almond oil, or any natural oil. It's really essential."

- **Sexy Feet.** Kris, a genuine olive oil lover, swears by olive oil for making her feet soft. "On an evening when you can soak your feet," she says, she does it, and she goes the whole 9 yards. "I rub olive oil to treat rough skin, then put on some thick socks. You can leave that on overnight. For a real soft foot treatment, soak those feet in vinegar first, then rub with olive oil and your feet will be baby soft."

TUB TIME

Bathing with olive oil is nothing new. Centuries ago, the Romans and the Egyptians used olive oil for moisturizing during and after tub time. By the nineteenth century, bathing for pleasure was a popular pastime in Europe and the word "spa" was created.

Some people claim that using a few drops of olive oil in a bath is a great natural moisturizer. But note, if you are prone to bladder infections or vaginal infections, contact your doctor before you take a dip and ask for a thumbs-up on using soothing olive oil combined with natural essential oils. (If it isn't recommended or if you don't have a bathtub, try plan B: Take a shower and use ready-made soaps with olive oil and essential oils.)

For best results, follow these suggestions straight from aromatherapy experts: Put specific essential oils on the skin before getting into the bath, light a scented candle or two for a sensual effect, and indulge in a cup of calming chamomile tea while you soak and beautify yourself.

Olive Oil and Scented Bath	Benefit	Essential Oil
Wake-up	Invigorates	Peppermint, rosemary
Foot soak	Relieves tired feet and athlete's foot	Witch hazel, tea tree
Aches	Relieves muscle soreness	Eucalyptus, lemon
De-stress	Relieves stress	Chamomile, orange
Insomnia	Promotes sleep	Lavender, chamomile

Using olive oil at home to pamper yourself is one thing, but traveling to a luxury spa and being pampered with olive oil is heaven—or it seems to be.

At the Napa Valley Lodge, California, the spa offers one beauty treatment, "Olive You." This is a massage/scalp and hair/foot treatment. The online description reads: "Your whole body, skin, hair and feet are cared for in this popular treatment. Your feet are scrubbed with olive oil, apricot kernels and peppermint oil and snugly wrapped to open the pores. Then we hydrate your feet with soothing balm . . . Finish with a grape seed/olive oil massage." The cost: $150 for a 90-minute treatment.

Or, at Carneros Inn in Napa, you can indulge in an "orchard olive stone and honeydew exfoliation. A unique exfoliation of warm crushed olive stones mixed with our native Carneros olive oil, followed by a luxurious massage with a rich honeydew body cream." The cost: $100 for a 45-minute treatment.

Now that you've got olive oil beauty secrets down, from head to toe, it's time to meet the real live people behind this liquid gold and the people who travel on the olive oil trail. We'll talk one-on-one with some unique people who make olive oil, as well as with folks who travel thousands of miles, to Sonoma, California, and Tuscany, Italy, to tour and taste olive oils.

THE GOLDEN SECRETS TO REMEMBER

✓ Olive oil–based ready-made products include bath oils, body gels, hand lotions, and shampoos.

✓ It takes special people to make special olive oil beauty products for people to enjoy.

✓ Olive oil from the bottle can condition your hair and skin—in or out of the tub—and be used to soften your body from your elbows to your feet.

✓ Remember, team olive oil with fragrant essential oils to double the effect and get health benefits, too.

✓ Olive oil treatments at luxury spas can be a treat to your senses.

CHAPTER

1 6

Olive Oil Producers, Tasting Bars, and Tours

Good oil, like good wine, is a gift from the gods.
—George Ellwanger[1]

During the research and writing of this book, it was fall, in the height of harvest season. Also, September 23 is the day celebrated for the olive tree. As a Libra, born on October 6, this is my favorite time of year. I can attest, however, that many olive oil producers were not favorable, at first, to my calls when I contacted them. I felt like a pesky intruder barging in at the wrong time, right place. For example, when I asked one woman the question "Which olive ranch is the largest in California?" she snapped, "Count the trees." But I pondered, "There has to be an easier way to determine which olive oil producers are successful." So, I put on my reading glasses and did my homework, both at home and at the olive oil orchards. (Just kidding.)

I soon discovered many of the olive oil producers and the manufacturers of olive oil–based products resided in Northern California, my home. And, many of them extended a warm Indian Summer welcome to me despite their grueling schedule to tend to their early or late harvest of olive oil.

EARLY AND LATE OLIVE HARVESTS

Fall Harvest Olive Oil: Olives reach their full size in the fall but may not fully ripen from green to black until late winter. Green olives have slightly less oil and more bitterness and can be higher in disease-fighting polyphenols. The oil tends to be more pricey because it takes more olives to make one bottle.

Many people like the peppery and bitter qualities of early-harvest oil. I like the former but pass on the latter, although it may just take a while to savor it, like getting used to goldenseal tea. Flavor notes of *astringent, grass, green, green leaf,* and *pungent* are used to describe early-harvest oils. Because of the higher polyphenols and antioxidants, early-harvest oils often have a longer shelf life and are blended with late-harvest oils to improve their shorter shelf life.

Winter Harvest Olive Oil: The fruit is picked black and ripe. The fruit may have a little more oil, but waiting to harvest it is risky business because as the days get shorter, the longer nights rev up the risk of the fruit being damaged by unwanted frost.

Late-harvest or "winter," fruit is naturally more ripe, so like other ripe fruit (think of a banana sitting on top of your refrigerator one day too many), it has a light, mellow taste with little bitterness and more floral flavors. Flavor notes of *apple, banana, buttery, fruity, melon, peach, perfumy, rotund, soave,* and *sweet* are often used.

Spring Harvest Olive Oil: Early March through late April is the last time to pick and press olives before the next season rolls around. These olives are ripe with a capital "R" and black on black all the way through to the pit. Olive oil from this season is the most delicate and "buttery sweet" available, dubbed "Limited Release" by California's Sciabica family due to its scarcity.

(*Source: The Olive Oil Source* and Sciabica.)

THE PRODUCERS

As I sit in my Northern California study, I confess that it didn't seem practical to book a flight to Europe and count the trees or acres to determine which producers are yielding the most olive oil. That would be a job in itself. And, in years to come, the number of trees and acres will change, from estate to estate, just as they do in California. But one man did do the legwork worldwide, so to speak. Charles Quest-Ritson provides impressive statistics about producers of olive oil in his book *Olive Oil.* The numbers will give you an idea. Here, take a look:

- **Spain.** Spain is touted as the largest olive-producing country worldwide. "It has more than 300 million olive trees covering more than five million acres, 92 percent of which are grown for olive oil," notes Quest-Ritson. Also, Jaen province produces a large percentage, and Martos is important. It claims to be the "World Capital of olive oil."[2]
- **Italy.** This country produces approximately 555,000 to 777,000 tons on a yearly basis. Nearly half of the total comes from Puglia, in southern Italy. Calabria, Sicily, and Campania follow.[3]
- **Greece.** These days, the total region planted with olives, says Quest-Ritson, is more than 2.4 million acres, with about 150 million olive trees, 2,800 mills, and more than 100 olive cultivars. What's more, Greece makes about 440,000 tons of oil each year.[4]

WIDESPREAD OLIVE APPEAL

While Spain, Italy, and Greece are known as the front-runners of olive oil production, other countries around the world are not ignoring olive oil. In China to Northern California, olive oil producers are showing enthusiasm with their orchards, mills, and olive oil.

Asian countries, for example, are paying attention to olive oil. Olive Connexions International boasts of 10,000 trees in Kunming, Yunnan, on its Web site. "There is a vast business potential for olive oil and its products in China . . . Local consumers, especially in the five Economic Zones and Beijing, Shanghai, Shenzhen and Hong Kong, are starting to switch to olive oil. Kunming, now an international expatriate hub, and the NW regions which have traditionally purchased olive oil from Turkey, are other local market possibilities."

Northern California is also becoming popular with the olive oil industry, with olive oil estates, tours, and tastings.

It is a competitive olive oil world, I learned. As a devout and serious dog person who used to breed Labrador retrievers and is now owned by two purebred Brittanys, I understand the ranking of and awards for dogs. It is similar in the world of olive oils. There are award-winning oils, judges, and tastings, and, well, olive oils can be ranked just like show dogs in a national or international show ring.

California Olive Oil—In Perspective

Paul Vossen of the University of California, Davis, has a handle on the California olive oil industry. Here's his outlook on California, which is the only state with significant production:

In 2006, California produced an estimated 400,000 gallons of olive oil, which is only 0.06% of the world's olive oil and less than 1% of the USA's domestic consumption of about 60 million gallons. . . .

Most of the 10,200 estimated acres of olive oil orchards in California have been planted in the last ten years; about 40% in just the last two years. Most of the older orchards that went in at the start of the gourmet olive oil resurgence in the late 1980s and early 1990s were planted in coastal counties. They are growing primarily Italian cultivars such as Frantoio, Leccino, Maurino, and Pendolino. Most of the newest plantings are located in the Central Valley with the varieties Arbequina, Arbosana, and Koroneiki. . . . When the currently planted acreage in California comes into bearing over the next 3–5 years, the state will be producing 1 million gallons of olive oil per year.

California's olive oils, as defined by flavor and style, have been closely associated with variety, harvest maturity, and processing technique. Many examples of California olive oils produced in the coastal counties, the Sierra foothills, and in Central Valley orchards have won awards internationally.

OLIVE OIL TASTING SMARTS

Here are several common terms you will hear aficionados use when judging the flavor of an olive oil.

Good Stuff	Bad Stuff
Almond: nutty	Bitter: good in moderation, but bad if overwhelming
Bitter: preferred trait of olive oils; often from green olives	Dirty: retains the unpleasant odor and flavor of its vegetable water, with which it remained in contact too long after pressing
Fresh: good aroma, fruity	Earthy: a musty humid odor from being pressed from unwashed, muddy olives
Grass: grass-like taste, common in green olives or those crushed with leaves and twigs	Flat: no aroma, tasteless
Green: young, fresh, fruity	Frozen: made from olives that weathered freezing temperatures; unpleasant odor
Peppery: a peppery bite in the back of the throat that causes a cough	Greasy: a grease flavor
Pungent: a burning sensation in the throat	Musty: moldy taste from being stored too long before pressing
Sweet: not bitter or pungent; common in mellow oils	Rancid: old; has begun to oxidize because of exposure to light or air

Source: John Deane, M.D.

OLIVE OIL TOUR DIARY: FORCES OF NATURE IN THE GOLDEN STATE

DAY ONE

As luck would have it, Murphy's Law is haunting me on November 28. As a resident of South Lake Tahoe, I shouldn't be surprised that Mother Nature would hinder our planned trip to "oliveland"—just three and a half hours away. A snowstorm is on its way, and it's wreaking havoc on our schedule to go to The Olive Press, Round Pond, B.R. Cohn, and Frantoio's. Well, we will visit all four hot olive oil spots—but not on the designated timetable.

One day late, at 4:10 P.M., my best friend, Kim Barrow, my younger brother, Bruce, and my two fun-loving Brittanys arrive intact near Round Pond in Rutherford, California. No snow in sight. I see a breathtaking Mediterranean type of terrain. The temperature is mild outdoors at the olive mill where oil is extracted from picked olives for Round Pond, a family-owned business that also makes vinegars and wines.

Amid the olive trees and European landscape, this mill sitting in Napa Valley is picture-perfect to me, a native of the Bay Area still trying to adapt to cold mountain weather, I think as I introduce myself to Jill Jackson, Round Hill's gracious tour director, who gives us a tour of the Rutherford oil mill.

She explains that Miles and Ryan MacDonnell, the owners, live on the premises, with some 2,100 trees in their 12-acre orchard. I am envious. It is so different from my mountain lifestyle, with pine trees surrounding my cabin, which sits a few blocks from Lake Tahoe. I feel like I am in another country—a European place.

Jackson shows us two of the mills. One has granite wheels to crush the olives. These are the best to play up the mellow Spanish-style oils. The other is a hammer mill to mince the olives into a pulp, best for Italian-style oils. Also, our tour guide emphasizes, time is of the essence—48 hours is the time for picking and crushing. No longer. This isn't vinegar; it's artisanal olive oil.

Inside a small room, Kim and I follow Jackson, who has an elegant table laid out for us, her two olive oil–tasting guests. A variety of olive oils are sitting in front of us surrounded by good-for-you edibles such as leafy lettuce, cheese, French bread, and red wine vinegar. Kim is bold and tastes each and every olive oil—the way it's supposed to be done. I make myself a salad and splash vinegar and olive oil on it. Not the right way to taste and judge, but it works for me. We thank our hostess and leave, realizing that olive oil is a serious business and there is a time to harvest and a time to reap. And our tour would have been longer if we had been on time, I think to myself.

It is back on the road, this time to Mill Valley. I have a 7:30 P.M. interview with Dr. Roberto Zecca, owner of Frantoio's Restaurant and the former president of the California Olive Oil Council. Once at the location, we check in at the Holiday Inn Express, chosen for its convenience and pet-friendly policy. (Rome, Italy, also has a pooch-friendly Holiday Inn, I recall.)

I choose to go solo for my interview. As I walk toward the restaurant, which boasts a terra-cotta–toned exterior, I fantasize I am in Italy, a place I will go to one day. Inside, I am told by the hostess that Dr. Zecca had a family emergency and therefore won't be able to make our interview date. Disappointed, I gaze around me and admire the high ceilings, stone floors, and built-in booths. I don't want to leave. Then, the general manager comes to my rescue.

I am whisked off to my own booth with a full view of the oakwood-fired oven. To the left of me, I also get to view Frantoio's state-of-the-art olive press—behind a gigantic piece of glass at the back of the busy restaurant. It has huge granite wheels, used to grind the olives to paste. This particular night, the press is down. (The olive press has since been replaced by a horizontal decanter centrifuge.) Still, I get a tour (and you can get a virtual one at www.frantoio.com) and am impressed that the restaurant makes its own extra virgin olive oil on-site. Plus, I later discover, Frantoio also provides custom presses for more than two dozen clients. It's unique, and so is the house-made extra virgin olive oil used in all of its dishes.

The menu boasts seasonal Tuscan delights using local produce and cheeses. As a vegan, I select the margherita brick-oven pizza, made with San Marzano tomatoes, mozzarella, basil, and extra virgin olive oil. As I sip chamomile tea, I dip homemade bread (with olives) into freshly made extra virgin olive oil. (Yes, for me, this is an adventure.)

Then, chef Duilio Valenti, a 30-something friendly man from Milan, pays a visit to my table. Not only are the pizza and service delightful, the ambiance is warm, casual, and comfortable.

Once I make my way back to the hotel, I am greeted by Kim, Bruce, and my two dogs. They ordered in from Frantoio's menu and I get a taste of more Italian cuisine: tortelloni filled with Pino's fresh ricotta and swiss chard with walnut sauce and olio novella, as well as more homemade bread. For dessert, Torre di Chioccolato, we indulge in a moist Valrhona chocolate cake tower. We are content with the chef's culinary skills.

DAY TWO

While my trip to the Valley of the Moon is an unforgettable one, it by no means is unique. Countless people visit olive oil spots, just like the two characters in the film *Sideways*, who go on a wine-tasting road trip.

I admit, due to the snowstorm, we are a day late arriving at The Olive Press. Still, we do get to experience another olive oil tasting. Olive oil experts will tell you that olive oil must be tasted to be "fully understood and appreciated." Think of wine or coffee aficionados. It takes practice and a knack to be able to differentiate a fine Chardonnay or delicious cup of java.

So, "How will I lose my inhibitions and taste the olive oils at The Olive Press?" I ponder. I rehearse the scenario: Pour a small amount of olive oil into a small cup. (But note, if you are at a tasting bar, this is often already done for you.) Place the cup in the palm of your hand and cover it with your fingers to warm it. After a minute or two, place the cup under your nose to appreciate the aroma of the oil.

I feel too shy to pretend to be Hannibal Lector (from the scene in the film *Silence of the Lambs* where he makes a frightening sucking noise with his mouth) or a veteran judge, so I invite my extroverted friend Jim Berkland, a geologist and longtime resident of Glen Ellen, known for its wineries, to show us the way to The Olive Press and step up to the cup, so to speak. And he did.

It is show time. While I had heard and read about the process, I watch it again take place in front of me. I view Berkland place a small amount of oil on his lower lip and, with the tip of his tongue, taste the oil for its degree of sweetness. Then, using the sides of his tongue, he sips the oil and tastes for spiciness. (I decide I will do the dip-my-bread-into-olive-oil tasting method in the privacy of my own home, in front of my nonjudgmental dogs and cat.)

The last stop is at B.R. Cohn Olive Oil Company in Glen Ellen. Because we are late, our tour has been cancelled. However, I do manage to come home with a Baronessa Cali Oliva Spa Viaggio Travel Set with extracts of Italian olive oil and a bar of Cali olive oil–based soap. And, for some reason, that makes everything all right, because I know I'll be able to pamper myself at home with the natural beauty products from my tour to where olives are blessed once a year.

Note to self: When a snowstorm threatens, go with the flow on an olive oil tasting tour, because you never know what you're going to get. Then again, one olive oil enthusiast got to visit both Napa Valley and Tuscany, and got the best of both worlds. . . .

Olive Alive

The olive trees are here, for sure,
And oh, those trees bring happiness
With olive oil that's mighty pure
For those who find The Olive Press.

The oval leaves of bluish green
Remain alive the whole year long,
And so they grace our country scene,
Although sometimes the trees go wrong.

That's when the ripened olives drop
Unharvested to coat the ground;
And then you may just need a mop,
Or watch your step when you're around.

But olive fruit, when treated right,
Gives salads just a touch of class;
And olives, stuffed, provide delight
When gracing your martini glass.

So olive trees have had their place
In Bible times, as well as now;
They've served to time the human race,
And now 'tis time to take their "bough."
—Jim Berkland
Glen Ellen, California

Tuscany's Trees to
Napa's Olives

Remember the Garden Lady, who gives her dog olive oil in his chow? She and her husband have had the fortunate delight to taste olive oil in Italy and Northern California. When she turned 50 (in 2000), she, C.L. Fornari, and her husband, Dan, went to Tuscany to celebrate. C.L. writes:

> Everywhere we went we tasted olive oil. A high point of the trip was walking the Cinque Terre, with olive trees growing on the steep hill to one side and the ocean on the other. We returned with several bottles of olive oil, and since then it has been a tradition to give olive oil as one of our New Year's gifts.
>
> There is no more beautiful and pastoral area than Tuscany. The gently rolling hills display whatever crop is being grown, be it sunflowers or olive trees. The light silver-green color of the olive leaves and the neatly spaced rows of trees that stretch over the hillsides are especially beautiful next to the terra-cotta and burnt sienna colors of the Northern Italian land. One of the many memories that I treasure from this trip is a trip to Venzano, a nursery and garden in Tuscany. En route, we stopped on the side of the road and got out of the car to admire the fields and olive groves. The only sound we heard was the clanking of the distant bells on the sheep in the fields. How rare that is in today's world—to only hear the sound of sheep's bells.
>
> When in Tuscany we were told that the traditional way to test olive oil is to pour some into the palm of your hand and smell it. It should smell fruity and very much of olives. Next, lick it off your palm—the freshest oil will be peppery, and the best will taste as fruity as it smells. In the stores for tourists, they offer small cubes of bread to soak up the oil for tasting, of course, and they often encourage people to start by tasting the blandest oils, working up to the strongest and most spicy. Dan and myself passed the watery oils by and went straight for the strongest stuff: why take in calories with little body and flavor?

Several years later, Dan and C.L. went to the wine country in Northern California. In November, with another couple—both couples celebrating their wedding anniversaries—they stayed at the Beltane Ranch, a historic Sonoma Valley bed and breakfast inn where they grow olives for oil. They tasted olive oils at many places in both Napa and Sonoma counties. Says C.L.:

> We set off in search of Katz and Company winding our way through a fairly industrial section of Napa to what seemed to be an office park. The woman explained that they had closed the Napa tasting room some years ago but she was happy to share their olive oil with us in the middle of the office/storeroom. The owner graciously offered us tastes. We tasted all the "Kitchen Line" offerings, and our favorite by far was the one they called "December Oil"—it is the first, fresh pressing of the season, so it is full of the most peppery olive flavor. That year we ordered "December Oil" Katz and Company for everyone on our New Year's list, and this year I did the same.
>
> The fact remains, there is an art to tasting olive oil, and who better to describe it than an olive oil farmer in Italy. . . .

LIKE AN ITALIAN

"It's up to an official tasters panel to determine the goodness of the oil in a sort of numerical range according to its flavor. But there is nothing to prevent you from personally doing this test much to your delight and satisfaction. Taste is rather subjective," notes olive oil farmer Antonio of Umbria, Italy. Here, take a look at his hands-on olive oil tasting tips:

- The test results will be better if you have not eaten for an hour and not smoked for 30 minutes.
- Take care to cleanse your palate with some water and a piece of bread before each tasting.
- Put a small amount of each of the different oils in different transparent glass bowls to examine their colors.
- Swirl the oil around in the bowl, warming it with your hands (so it can rise above room temperature) and evaluate the oil's fluidity.
- Inhale deeply to note the intensity of the bouquet.

- Take some drops in your mouth and softly put your tongue to your palate to get the first flavors.
- Take a more substantial draught of the oil (a teaspoon), mixing it with air to help release the flavors. Before swallowing, keep it in your mouth for 20 seconds to gradually enjoy the taste.
- Enjoy the intensity of the aftertaste.

I can tell you, though, as an unbiased individual who is a newbie at tasting olive oils, that while experiencing the different olive oils you will wonder, "How can I use this type in my cooking?" According to the Olive Press experts, there are three distinct categories of extra virgin olive oils:

- *Mild*: Buttery, sweet. Perfect with broiled and grilled fish, hot and cold vegetable soups, sauces without garlic, cooked and steamed vegetables, meat and carpaccio, and cheeses.
- *Fruity*: "Olivey," that is, green (tasting of grass, leaves, or fruit) or ripe. Complements grilled meat and vegetables, pasta, bruschetta without garlic, sauces with garlic, and milder cheeses.
- *Fruity-pungent*: Spicy, peppery (perceived in throat). Perfectly complements traditional, rustic dishes such as bruschetta with garlic, pasta e fagioli (pasta and beans), ribollita (vegetable-and-bread soup), and panzella (tomato-and-bread salad).

AN OLIVE OIL TOUR DE FORCE

While going to Umbria to taste olive oil is my dream, it isn't necessary to fly thousands of miles to do so. But some people in the world will trek far enough to get the good stuff. Sara Conley, an olive oil enthusiast, recalls an exciting adventure that she shared with her boyfriend, Robert A. Salitore II. She told me, "We flew from O'Hare International to San Luis Obispo County airport via L.A. on Thursday, November 30. We were lucky enough to stay in the little white cottage on the ranch as guests. Rob and I weren't afraid to try the oil right after pressing because the Pasolivo oil is so flavorful to begin with, and we are such huge fans, we knew it would be right up our alley."

Rob vividly recollects the unforgettable olive oil touring adventure at Paso Robles, California, on December 1, 2006. . . .

On this day a group of us who love the peppery, green good-ness of Pasolivo are assembled to see how it all happens. Dressed in boots and work clothes, we've come to see the oil made from start to finish.

Joeli Yaguda leads us out into the olive orchard. We get the history of the ranch on the way over and her love for the place shines through. Then, we arrive at our row of trees, with their silvery green leaves and limbs drooping with ripe olives. Each of the 17 of us either straps a bucket to the front of our chest or carries one by hand. We are shown by the ranch manager how to glide one hand down the limb and direct the olives into the bucket. He gets every olive off in one clean motion. He's a pro.

Then, we're off into the trees. We have to keep to the low hangers because no ladders are allowed. We strip olives from the tree with both hands while hearing the thump, thump, thump as they hit the bottom of the bucket. We're told to pick all of the olives, green and black alike. It seems when you harvest an olive tree you harvest them all, ripe or not so ripe.

Everyone in the group is getting into the process and after an hour we picked 308 pounds. We beat the group who had visited the day before and a group of 2nd graders from the previous week. We've all warmed up substantially, taken off our outer layers, and gaze at our collection as workers all around us continue climbing trees and harvesting. They've been there since 5 A.M. and will continue working into the night. The entire harvest takes two weeks of 12 hour days and we were lucky enough to experience it.

Back at the tasting room and mill we sit down for a sensory analysis. We are each served three olive oils blindly. We pick up the glass to warm it, then lift our hand to let the aroma surround our nose. We take in the fruity, grass smell and then lift the glass, one by one, to our lips. Amazing.

Back out in the mill room, the olives we've harvested are getting a bath. Afterward they ride up a conveyor and inside to the mill, which whirrs and whirrs without stopping. Soon I'm brought over to a barrel which is being fed a stream of neon green liquid from an overhead pipe. This is olive oil made from olives that I harvested with my own hands hours before. I'm given a small pitcher which I dip under the liquid. I insert a funnel into a small bottle and pour from the pitcher the freshest olive oil I could ever imagine. Next comes a stopper and a label, and we're in business. I feel so connected to the oil, and wish I had a hand in making all of the food and wine I consume. Modern life really doesn't afford us that opportunity, but I am grateful for the chance to go from olive to oil with my very own hands.

As you can see, olive oil producers, tasting bars, and tours can be found in Northern and Southern California as well as in Italy—the place I plan to go one day, especially now that I am learning to appreciate olives and olive oil.

In fact, Gloria Cappelli and her partner, Marcel C. Gordon, described to me their vacation rental. Here, let her paint the postcard-perfect picture for you if you're looking for a holiday home in Tuscany. . . .

Casina di Rosa is an old 19th century village house; my great-grandparents built it over 100 years ago. It never left the family, and in 2003 when we had to face the choice of selling or doing something with it, wince it had been empty for quite a while, we decided to try and rent it by the week to foreign guests. I am from the village, Civtella Marittima. Both my parents were also from the village. I am very fond of the area, which is called Upper Maremma and is part of Tuscany. The house is very tiny, only 400 square feet. There are four rooms: a kitchen with the old fireplace which we kept in the renovation, the bedroom, a sitting room which we have equipped with guidebooks and books about olive oil, the bathroom. By the main entrance there is a small patio with two chairs to enjoy the morning sun and watch the village life go by.

Siena is one of the most beautiful cities in Tuscany. Grosseto is the capital of the Maremma, a subregion of Tuscany, scarcely populated by Italian standards. The house is in the village, so there are other stone houses, little streets, and great views over the valley, as the village is on the top of a hill. Just walk five minutes and you will find as many olive trees as you wish.

My father has olive groves all around the village. When I am available I take guests to our fields, otherwise Carlo Barbieri takes them to Podere Vignali where it is like *Under the Tuscan Sun*, maybe better. In small villages reaching the farmed countryside is so easy that it is like living in the countryside itself.

For more information, log onto http://www.casinadirosa.it/.

A DAY IN A LIFE WITH OLIVE OIL

Whether you live in Chicago, Tuscany, or Lake Tahoe, olive oil—and its products—can lure you to travel to see what the olive oil world is all about. Take a look at my new daily agenda, which revolves around the healing powers of oil. In the cold, dry mountain winter climate of Lake Tahoe, I don't know how I survived without it.

8:00 A.M.: Spray the frying pan with extra virgin olive oil before I scramble two eggs. Gemma Sciabica taught me this trick, and it works like a charm. No more brown, toasty eggs on my plate.

8:30 A.M.: Shower with olive oil–based soap (rosemary/sage); wash hair with olive oil–based shampoo and crème rinse.

8:45 A.M.: Massage extra virgin olive oil into my feet and hands.

9:00 A.M.: Too cold to shampoo the dogs, so I put a drop of extra virgin olive oil on Simon's back and brush him thoroughly. Ditto for Seth.

10:00 A.M.: Water houseplants in the dining room and spritz with a mixture of water and olive oil.

Noon: Warm up French bread in the microwave along with a small bowl of flavored olive oil. Toss together a salad of greens, tuna, tomatoes, olive oil, and red wine vinegar.

1:00 P.M.: Use olive oil and lemon to dust the desk and living room table in an attempt to remove teacup rings.

5:00 P.M.: Order a vegetarian pizza: spinach, tomatoes, mushrooms, and olives.

5:30 P.M.: Bring in wood for the fire. Wash my hands and rub olive oil moisturizing hand lotion on my cuticles after making the fire.

9:00 P.M.: Give myself a pedicure. After the polish has dried, I apply olive oil generously to the bottoms of my feet and put on fresh socks for the rest of the evening.

10:00 P.M.: Wipe out both Brittanys' ear canals with extra virgin olive oil. They're going to the vet tomorrow, and I want them to be clean for the technician.

11:00 P.M.: Take a primose oil gelcap and hope that it will help deal with post-menopausal woes.

Midnight: Take a quick glance at *The Healing Powers of Olive Oil* to find news ways I can use versatile, all-natural olive oil (and other oils) to make my life easier and more bearable in the mountains.

Now that you know everything good you wanted to know about olive oil but were afraid to ask, let's take a close-up and personal look at the downside (unfortunately, not even olive oil is 100 percent perfect) of this healing liquid.

The Golden Secrets to Remember

- ✓ Harvest season is from fall to late winter, and olive oil can vary in taste depending on the time of year it is made.
- ✓ Spain, Italy, and Greece are the regions where olive oil production is most prevalent, but olive oil producers exist around the globe.
- ✓ People use a variety of terms, such as "bitter" and "flat," when judging the flavor of an olive oil.
- ✓ Northern California is gaining in popularity as a place where award-winning olive oils are produced; tours and tasting bars are very vogue.
- ✓ Olive oil enthusiasts, much like wine lovers, will travel to Tuscany and Northern California to tour, taste, and bring home artisanal olive oils.
- ✓ While the Golden State's olives are grown in Northern California, central California also has its place in the olive oil world.
- ✓ In the twenty-first century, you don't have to travel anywhere to indulge in olive oil and its array of products. Olive oil is everywhere, and you can use it for cooking, bathing, cleaning, beauty, pet care, and so much more, just like in ancient biblical times.

Olive Oil Is Not for Everyone: Some Bitter Views

England and the English, as a rule they will refuse even to sample a foreign dish, they regard such things as garlic and olive oil with disgust, life is unliveable to them unless they have tea and puddings.
—George Orwell[1]

Speaking of olive oil aficionados, there are some people who cannot and will not tolerate the golden liquid. While olive oil can be used both inside and outside the body, some people insist it causes problems.

Taking a tablespoon or two of olive oil solo on a daily basis (like Professor Seth Roberts did to maintain his weight loss) may not be the perfect remedy for everyone. There are people who have turned to olive oil for good health and other uses, but there are many others who have made an oil change or are turned off by olive oil for different reasons. Here's why.

TOO MUCH OF A GOOD THING

Does all this good news about olive oil nudge you to run, not walk, to your nearest supermarket, health food store, or online retailer for a bottle of the golden liquid? If so, remember that olive oil and other oils are not calorie-free. One tablespoon of the elixir with healing powers boasts 120 calories, give or take a few. That means, calorie-wise, you can't pour the golden liquid on everything from pasta and potatoes to dipping bread and bagels. Doing so can cause a good thing to have weighty results. Translation: It isn't difficult to pack on un-wanted pounds fast if you overdo it with olive oil, or with any food that packs calories—"good" fat or not. But even if you don't go over-board, you may run into another problem.

SENSITIVITY TO OLIVE OIL

One woman, for example, claims her boyfriend, a no-nonsense globe-trotter, enjoys olive oil–based recipes in his travels to places like Greece and Spain. Unfortunately, within 30 minutes, the adventurous foodie ends up in the restroom for longer than he'd prefer.

According to John Deane, M.D., "Sensitivity to olive oil is rare but certainly possible. If the oil cannot be absorbed for some reason, it will act as a cathartic. Extra virgin olive oil is not processed, the olives are simply ground up and the oil removed by pressing or spinning in a centrifuge."

He adds, "The type of olives used for oil production may contain as much as 20% of their weight in oil. The larger varieties grown for pick-ling and brining often have as little as 5% oil, so it is not surprising that eating olives doesn't cause the same problem."

BAKING BLUNDERS

Gemma Sciabica, a nutrition-savvy woman and the author of four cookbooks, guarantees that olive oil can and does work in baking, even in double-layer chocolate cakes and pie crusts for your favorite apples. Note to self: I will try both.

But, some folks don't have pleasant experiences with olive oil in their baking adventures. A Midwest writer, for one, explains that she loves olive oil. "However, olive oil only goes so far. For my birthday, my husband made me a dark chocolate cake and, not being a baker, he didn't even notice the difference between the two oils (canola and olive) and the cake was unbearable; although it was moist, it had this thick, distinct olive oily taste that overpowered the dark chocolate. But I was just so happy for the effort I barely noticed. The next day, the cake found its way to the Dumpster."

Another fellow writer recalls, "The only olive oil story I have is that it put me in the doghouse. My girlfriend was making last-minute pumpkin bread for a party and got mad at me when I tried to use olive oil in place of vegetable oil. (I told her we had oil when she was out shopping.)"

So, what was the end result? "My girlfriend wouldn't let me use the olive oil and sent the first person to arrive at our party to the store to buy canola oil. Funny, she usually enjoys olive oil, but for some reason felt this olive oil discrimination and guest imposition was worth it. The pumpkin bread has so much sugar in it that I'm pretty sure Brylcreem would have worked in place of the oil," adds the disgruntled boyfriend, who believes olive oil would have sufficed. And that's not all . . .

CAN OLIVE OIL GO BAD?

Since I'm on a roll regarding worst-case-scenario olive oil stories, I might as well include my own personal experience. Blame it on my lack of knowledge about cooking and storing cooking oils. In my thirties, a friend of mine was moving to Los Angeles. In return, I got to stock my pantry with lots of his kitchen cupboard goodies—including a bottle of olive oil.

One night, I got the desire to whip up a pasta dish. I used all fresh vegetables and pasta. Then, I tossed it with the olive oil. (Remember, I knew nothing at all about the shelf life of oils.) So, I didn't think twice about its longevity, assuming it was like a good wine, which gets better as it ages, right? One hour later: I was dead wrong. In the bathroom, I grew very sick. The bottom line: The olive oil was rancid, and I will never forget it. I tossed it for good.

So, how long does olive oil last, anyhow? You'll find different answers to this question. It isn't cut-and-dried as for vinegar, which does get better with age. The consensus is, store it in a cool, dark place. Also, keep it away from heat. But note: Some types of oils, such as flavored oils, should be refrigerated.

While it would be great if all oils could last for one year, I logged on to the olive oil storage questions page at the Spectrum Naturals Web site to find out if their products have an expiration or "best if used by" date. As they put it: "Refrigeration is not required for our oils, but it does keep them fresher for a longer period of time. We recommend refrigeration for all of Spectrum's culinary oils with the exception of our Coconut Oil, which is very stable due to the amount of saturated fat in the oil."

Then, since I have an assortment of olive oils in my pantry, I read further and learned the following:

- *Frequent Use:* If you use the oil frequently and will go through it quickly—within two months, for example—it's fine to leave it in a cool, dark place. Once opened, it's best to consume it within 60 days.
- *Extended Storage:* If you plan to use your oil infrequently, you may want to consider refrigerating it to extend its freshness and shelf life. Please note that many oils with a high monounsaturated fat content, such as olive oil, will partially solidify when refrigerated. This does not harm the oil, but it does make it inconvenient. To re-liquefy, simply allow the oil to return to room temperature.
- *The Details:* Proper storage is important for maintaining the integrity of the oils. Heat, oxygen, and light are the most common damaging elements for oils. The more natural an oil, the more protection it needs.

    Ideally, to safeguard the nutritive value and longevity of your oils, keep them in a cool (40°–72°), dark cupboard until opening. Then, store them in your refrigerator. Storage under these conditions provides a shelf life of 10 to 14 months for unrefined oils and 14 to 20 months for refined oils.

As you can see, the shelf life of an olive oil product depends on a variety of things, such as storage time, temperature, age, and container. I suggest you contact the manufacturer if you have any concerns rather than pull a stunt like I did and end up in the bathroom wishing you had the right knowledge about the shelf life of olive oil.

HARD TO SWALLOW

Statistics show that olive oil is growing in popularity. But that doesn't mean everyone can take a tablespoon (or two) per day like Dr. Seth Roberts to maintain his or her weight, dip his or her bread into the warm oil, or drizzle it on his or her salad. So, what do you do if you want the health benefits but can't bear to swallow this important food?

Olive leaf extract may be the answer for you. Yes, you can get condensed olive oil in tea, capsules, and other forms, and it may be easier for you to take. There are many health food stores that carry a variety of olive leaf extract products.

As time goes on, I predict that olive oil—and other healing oils— will be used in more kitchens around the globe. Not only is it part of a healthful Mediterranean diet (which is being put to work more and more for good health), but it has earned its good household name. Last and by no means least, in Chapter 18, "The Joy of Cooking with Olive Oil," I am pleased to share creative and nutritious cooking tips and recipes. Included are olive oil–based dishes, from such well-known chefs as Michel Stroot, former chef at California's Golden Door Spa, and Gemma Sciabica. These people, and others from olive oil associations nationwide, understand Mediterranean cuisine and stand behind the healthful liquid gold.

THE GOLDEN SECRETS TO REMEMBER

✓ Olive oil can be one person's best medicine and another individual's worst nightmare, depending on how it's used and the person who uses it.

✓ A sensitivity to olive oil—like a sensitivity to anything—can happen, but it isn't common.

✓ Pay attention to the "use by" date. You do not want to use olive oil that has expired.

✓ Olive oil and other oils can and are used in baking every day, and have been for years.

✓ Keep in mind that food chains across the nation—starting in New York—are banning unhealthy trans fats from muffins, cookies, and other baked goods, and replacing them with healthier oils.

CHAPTER

1 8

The Joy of Cooking with Olive Oil

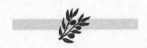

EVOO.

—Rachael Ray

World-renowned chef Mario Batali has said that "olive oil is as precious as gold." Television personality Rachael Ray, a *Food Network* regular, uses catchy phrases such as "EVOO" in reference to extra virgin olive oil. What's more, the word is that Ray's acronym, EVOO, is being added to the *Oxford American College Dictionary.*

It's no secret that chefs, on the little and big screens, in restaurants and their own kitchens, treasure olive oil, be it on the West Coast, East Coast, or Mediterranean basin.

The recipes in *The Healing Powers of Olive Oil* are created with fresh superfoods—nutrient-dense vegetables, fruits, grains, legumes, fish, poultry, and olive oil. Our wide array of dishes, provided by chefs from Europe and olive oil experts who have visited Spain, Italy, and Greece, contain a variety of oils—olive oil, flaxseed oil, canola oil, and herbal oils. Plus, good-for-you garlic, onions, and red wine and balsamic vinegars are often part of the recipes, too.

For best results, use the olive oil brand noted in each recipe. However, feel free to use your own brand or a brand without sodium (you want to keep unwanted pounds and high blood pressure at bay, whatever age you are). Or, if you are lean and have normal blood pressure, treat yourself to the wide collection of specialty flavored olive oils.

Before you begin, take a look at some tips for cooking with olive oil, which can help you make these recipes turn out fabulous. Olive oil and other oils teamed with health-boosting, good-for-you foods will not only keep your weight in check but may add years to your life. It was my intention to bring European flair to your kitchen, since not all of us can whisk away to Italy in a heartbeat. So, use a variety of these original, healthful, and delicious recipes perfect for a heart-healthy, anti-cancer, Mediterranean-style diet. If you're like me (a non-foodie), or if you are an adventurous foodie, you may wonder what took you so long to cook up an olive oil-based delight paired with healthful companion foods. It's a healthy romance with food that I, and you, can savor time after time year round.

THE WORLD OF OILS

So, what oils should you use in cooking? Roe Valenti, a veteran chef and caterer who cooks for herself, her family, and her friends, told me she likes to cook with only one oil—olive oil. When I asked her, "Why olive oil?" she had the answer.

"When I was a kid, my grandmother used to tell me, 'Don't ever use anything other than olive oil. It's good for you.' So olive oil was part of my daily diet. You know us Italians. We use olive oil for everything, from salads to pasta. Perhaps that's why our record for longevity is a good one."[1]

The only other oil she recommended is canola, to make your own salad dressing or to put in your water when you're going to boil pasta. "Aside from these uses, it's olive oil all the way. And it's funny, because when I go to a friend's house to make dinner they know they will get a healthy meal. But, when I say, 'I'm going to sauté the veggies first' the response is the same, 'You're going to sauté the food with oil?' I answer, 'Yes, with olive oil, there is no need to worry.' Then, after I get the taste from the olive oil combined into the food I'm cooking, that's it. Any other moisture I get is from wine, broth or water."[2]

Italians like Valenti love olive oil—but there are so many types of oil, as you know—including the wide world of flavored oils. Take a look and see how you can put to use the wonderful flavors of olive oil in your cooking.

OILS WITH HEART AND SOUL!

Oil	Flavor	Uses
Canola oil	Mild	All purpose for cooking, salads, baking
Extra virgin olive oil	Fruity, intense	Drizzling, salads, marinades, sauces, stews, soups
Virgin olive oil	Strong, but milder than EVOO	Grilling, sautéing, drizzling, salad dressings, marinades, stews, soups
Peanut oil	Intense	Stir-fries, sautéing
Olive oil	Mild	Baking, frying, grilling, sautéing
Light olive oil	Very mild	Baking, frying, grilling, sautéing
Basil olive oil	Fresh taste in pesto	Dipping, drizzling, vegetables, tomatoes, tomato-based sauces, Southeast Asian cuisine, soups, salads, pastas, stir-fries
Garlic-flavored olive oil	Zesty, added zip	Sautéing, vegetables, pasta
Jalapeño olive oil	Hot, peppery	Southwest dishes, eggs
Lemon-flavored olive oil	Tangy, light	Salads, fish, chicken
Lime-flavored olive oil	Tangy, light	Salads, fish
Orange-flavored olive oil	Tangy, light	Chicken, duck

Oil	Flavor	Uses
Oregano olive oil	Intense	Tomatoes, pizza, tomato-based sauces, pasta, dressings
Pepper olive oil	Hot, peppery	Sautéing, roasting, eggs, seafood, Southwest cuisine
Porcini olive oil	Sweet	Vegetable dishes
Rosemary olive oil	Strong, pungent	Roasted potatoes, eggplant, artichokes, asparagus, dressings, breads
Tangerine olive oil	Tangy, light	Salads, chicken

BASIC COOKING TIPS

Rely on the full flavor and versatility of olive oil to create dishes that satisfy everyone. From appetizers to entrées to desserts, olive oil can be a key ingredient in the preparation of meals. As with all ingredients, though, make sure you're using it right to get the most benefit. Just follow these savvy tips:

- As a general rule, cook with olive oil, but season or drizzle with extra virgin olive oil after the food is prepared.
- Serve a small dish of extra virgin olive oil at meals. Rather than using butter or margarine, dip bread or rolls in olive oil for a spectacular new taste.
- Deep-fry foods in light olive oil, and watch them turn golden brown.
- Enjoy garlic bread by brushing extra virgin olive oil on both halves of a split loaf of Italian or French bread. Sprinkle with chopped garlic or garlic powder, and broil until lightly browned.
- Baste turkey and chicken with extra virgin olive oil for extra flavor.

- Use extra virgin olive oil to replace the smoked meats and sausages that are typically used to flavor bean and pea soups.
- Sauté nuts in a little extra virgin olive oil for added flavor.
- For a tasty dessert, sauté bananas, apples, pears, or other fruits in light olive oil. Sprinkle with cinnamon and sugar, and serve.

(*Source:* North American Olive Oil Association.)

BOOSTING YOUR COOKING-SPRAY SMARTS

So, have you noticed that chefs often use spray oils? For instance, Michel Stroot, a former Golden Door Spa chef of 30 years, turns to oil in a spray bottle for some of his recipes.

"We use spray bottles to mist oil onto pans and food. This enables you to use less oil, reducing total fat in the dish," he notes in *The Golden Door Spa Cooks Light & Easy* (Gibbs Smith, 2005). While commercially available oil sprays are convenient, he prefers to use his own oils. He keeps two spray bottles near his cooking arena. He recommends filling one bottle with straight canola oil. Fill the other with a combo of 1 part olive oil and 3 parts canola oil. He also points out that canola oil is ideal for cooking because of its high smoking point. "You can raise the heat properly and brown your food," he says. But it's olive oil that adds the fabulous flavor, he adds. As a result, you can have the best of both worlds of oils.[3]

Note, however, that some people may prefer to use a store-bought oil spray. There are manufacturers who offer a wide collection of spray oils, from conventional to organic, as well as canola, grapeseed, and olive oils.

Q. Can spray oil be used at any heat?

A. Just like bottled oil, spray oils are best when used below their "smoke point," the temperature at which the oil begins to smoke. At this point, the oil releases unhealthy free radicals. Look on the side of the can for the recommended heat for the spray oil that you are using.

Q. What are the advantages of cooking with spray oils?

A. They're perfect partners for grilling, frying, and baking. A quick spray or two allows the fresh flavors of your ingredients to shine through, and prevents foods from sticking. And spray oils are a great way to cut calories, too. [The canola oils are cold-pressed, and the grapeseed oil is alcohol-extracted. No chlorofluorocarbons are used in the aerosol delivery system.]

Q. *How should I store spray oils?*
A. Properly stored per label instructions, they have a 2-year shelf life. Look for them in the cooking oil section.
(*Source:* Spectrum Naturals.)

On Top of Old Smoky Point of Oils

Here are six types of oils and their smoke points, according to John Deane, M.D.

Oil Type	Smoke–Point Temperature
Avocado	485°
Canola	400°
Extra virgin olive	420°
Grapeseed	485°
High-end and extra virgin olive	375°
Sesame	410°

ROME IN A BOTTLE

Speaking of storing olive oil, C. L. Fornari, aka "The Garden Lady," who has experienced tasting tours in Tuscany and gives her pooch olive oil, has more to say about how she preserves her olive oil in her kitchen. . . .

I keep the following objects right next to my stove: a jar of spatulas, strainers and wooden spoons, another filled only with pairs of scissors, and a third filled with potholders. In front of these are salt and pepper grinders and a dark green glass bottle of olive oil. I consider olive oil to be more important than the salt and pepper, and since I usually leave salt out of recipes and often leave the addition of pepper for when the dish hits the table, the olive oil is probably the most important ingredient on my kitchen counter.

I use a dark green bottle here because the light breaks down the oil when it's in a clear glass container. I have a fancy olive oil bottle with a nicely designed metal pouring spout, but the glass is clear so I seldom use it. I'll purchase one of the less expensive oils in a dark green bottle, or refill an empty bottle from a can of oil that is kept in my cool garage.

Ah, that reminds me: My husband's family are Italian Jews, from Rome. During the second World War Dan's father enlisted in the U.S. Army and worked in Army Counter Intelligence because he spoke several languages, but his mother's family went into hiding in the Italian countryside south of Rome. They were lucky enough to have land where they could raise their own food, as well as grapes and olives that could be traded for other things. After the war Dan's mother and father (not married during the war, but they were high school sweethearts) met up again and got married, and came to this country in the late 1940s. The land where his mother's family was in hiding is now in other hands, but continues to produce olive oil and wine. A cousin orders several large cans of oil from the owners each year and sells them to whomever is interested. Feeling a connection to that place and the olive trees on the farm, we always buy some.

LEARNING TO LOVE OLIVE OIL

I have read how olive oil lovers swear off butter and margarine and embrace olive oil as their fat of choice. I admit, it takes a while to get used to the change, just like when you switch to drinking tea instead of soda or eating dark chocolate instead of milk chocolate. But if you do it for 30 days, people say it will become habit. If you're wondering how to make the change, having a conversion chart may be helpful.

CONVERSION OF BUTTER TO OLIVE OIL

Butter	Olive Oil
1 teaspoon	¾ teaspoon
1 tablespoon	2¼ teaspoons
¼ cup	3 tablespoons
⅓ cup	¼ cup
½ cup	¼ cup + 2 tablespoons
⅔ cup	½ cup
¾ cup	½ cup + 1 tablespoon
1 cup	¾ cup

Source: The Olive Press

If you love chocolate, you can learn to love olive oil and get a double heart-healthy fix. Recently, I baked brownies. Okay, I didn't make them from scratch, but I did include three eggs (the kind with omega-3s), dark chocolate, fresh walnuts, whole wheat flour (I live in a high altitude), and extra virgin olive oil. Yes, they were tasty and, most likely, healthier than packaged brownies. Next, I will bake a cake with olive oil—such as The Olive Press Citrus Cake (and top it with fresh berries). It is included in the following five-day menu plan.

THE OLIVE OIL HEALTH-BOOSTING FIVE-DAY MENU PLAN

This five-day "California Diet" is based on a nutritious and slimming diet plan I created years ago. It is the way I eat now, too. But I have enhanced it with heart-healthy, irresistible Mediterranean dishes.

Day 1

Breakfast:
 1 serving oatmeal with low-fat milk and 1 tablespoon raisins
 1 orange
 Glorious Morning Muffin*
 1 boiled egg

Lunch:
 1 cup non-fat or low-fat yogurt
 ½ cup raw baby carrots with Golden State Olive Dip (Mix
  together ⅔ cup plain low-fat yogurt, ¼ cup finely minced red
  onion, 2 tablespoons sliced olives, 1 tablespoon minced fresh
  chives, and 1 tablespoon chopped fresh garlic.)
 Greek Salad*
 1 plain whole wheat bagel

Snack:
 Fresh fruit
 Herbal tea

Dinner:
 Simple Salmon*
 1 baked potato drizzled with flavored olive oil and diced tomatoes
 1 slice French bread dipped in olive oil
 1 glass red wine or herbal tea

Snack:
 Fresh fruit

Day 2

Breakfast:
 1 serving whole grain cereal
 1 cup skim or low-fat milk
 6 ounces fresh carrot or papaya juice

* Recipe can be found in Part 7, "Olive Oil Recipes."

Lunch:
Cioppino*
1 cup leafy spinach with red wine vinegar and olive oil dressing
1 slice French bread dipped in olive oil
1 cup non-fat or low-fat yogurt

Snack:
Fresh fruit

Dinner:
Summer Vegetable and Organic Tofu Tacos*
1 cup fresh fruit salad

Snack:
1 slice The Olive Press Citrus Cake*

Day 3

Breakfast:
2 eggs, scrambled in frying pan lightly sprayed with olive oil
Sweet Potato Biscuit*
6 ounces fresh juice

Lunch:
3 ounces tuna and ½ cup leafy spinach stuffed into a whole wheat
    pita pocket with ½ sliced tomato and alfalfa sprouts
8 ounces skim or low-fat milk

Snack:
Fresh fruit

Dinner:
Angel Hair Pasta with Diced Tomatoes, Edamame Beans, Basil,
    and Virgin Olive Oil*
Tossed green salad with vinegar dressing
1 cup broccoli or asparagus spears

Snack:
Fresh fruit

Day 4

Breakfast:
$\frac{1}{2}$ cup low-fat granola
$\frac{1}{2}$ cup skim milk
1 orange
Glorious Morning Muffin*

Lunch:
Open-faced grilled cheese sandwich with avocado and tomato
slices
1 cup gazpacho soup
1 cup fresh fruit salad

Snack:
Greek Salad*

Dinner:
Herbed Roast Turkey*
$\frac{1}{2}$ cup mashed potatoes
$\frac{1}{2}$ cup green vegetable drizzled with lemon olive oil

Snack:
$\frac{1}{2}$ cup vanilla ice cream drizzled with balsamic vinegar

Day 5

Breakfast:
Vegetable omelet (Sauté $\frac{1}{4}$ cup each broccoli, red onion, and red
bell pepper in 1 teaspoon olive oil for 5–10 minutes. Whisk
together 1 egg and 2 egg whites and pour over vegetables.
Sprinkle with Cheddar cheese before serving.)
$\frac{1}{2}$ cup skim or low-fat milk
6 ounces fresh juice

Lunch:
1 tomato slice and skim Mozzarella cheese grilled on whole grain
bagel half and drizzled with olive oil
1 apple
1 cup skim or low-fat milk

Snack:
> Fresh olives with Golden State Olive Dip (See Day 1 lunch for recipe.)

Dinner:
> Halibut with Caper Sauce*
> Golden Door Salad with Tonnata Dressing*
> 1 slice French bread drizzled with olive oil

Snack:
> Fresh fruit

Now that you've learned everything you wanted to know about olive oil but were afraid to ask, it's time to bring in recipes for your olive oil future, in Part 7, "Olive Oil Recipes."

THE GOLDEN SECRETS TO REMEMBER

✓ Mediterranean-type cooking includes nutrient-dense foods such as vegetables, fruits, grains, legumes, fish, poultry, and olive oil.

✓ There are countless olives oils to choose from when you are cooking, whether it is extra virgin olive oil, light olive oil, or flavored herb or citrus oils.

✓ Cooking sprays can help you be the best cook you can be.

✓ Storing your olive oils the right way will keep you and the people for whom you cook healthy and safe from oil that has expired.

✓ The Olive Oil Health-Boosting Five-Day Menu Plan is a sample of how you can incorporate heart-healthy and unforgettable olive oil–based recipes into your life—without going to Europe.

PART 7

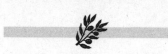

OLIVE OIL RECIPES

Olive Oil Bon Appétit!

Welcome to these original recipes for dozens of tasty delights, full of nutritious vegetables, fruits, fish, and poultry. These dishes, provided by chefs from around the country, contain a variety of healthy oils—but mostly olive oil and canola oil. Many of these recipes also use garlic, onions and herbs.

For best results, use the olive oil brand mentioned in each recipe. However, feel free to use your own brand or another type of oil (such as canola oil). But note, Italian cook and olive oil guru Gemma Sciabica recommends using health-promoting extra virgin olive oil for *all* recipes.

Before you get started, I want you to first take the olive oil quiz; discover epicurean enjoyment; and put to use must-have olive oil tips. Not only will you be eating a heart-healthy, anti-cancer Mediterranean-style diet, you'll be enjoying more taste and excitement in your meals as well as lifestyle for the rest of your life.

WHICH OLIVE OIL
IS RIGHT FOR YOU?

Olive oil judges from coast to coast and around the world recognize award-winning olive oils, but despite their awards, some of these oils may not be a suitable match for you and your lifestyle. For instance, if you don't like mushrooms, porcini olive oil may not be your cup of oil. You may love to cook, but extra virgin olive oil may not give you enough pizzazz. Like to bake but don't want to be stuck using only canola oil (one healthful oil) for your breads, cakes, and muffins? You may be limiting yourself with your oil of choice.

No matter what kind of oil lover you are, take this quiz to get to know your personality and your real taste in oil before you choose the oil(s) for you.

Oils for Life

What's your lifestyle? Take this short quiz to find out.

1. A typical morning for you includes:
    A. Family chaos, with the dog joining in.
    B. Breakfast in bed.
    C. A 2-mile run.
    D. Computer work.
    E. Brunch at an ethnic restaurant.

2. When you cook, you like to:
    A. Feed a fun-loving crowd.
    B. Feed a loving mate or friend who enjoys your meals.
    C. Make a meal to take on the run.
    D. Make a low-maintenance meal.
    E. Work in a kitchen chock-full of exotic treats.

3. Your idea of a perfect vacation is:
    A. Grabbing the family and visiting relatives.
    B. Going to a secluded park for a picnic.
    C. Hitting the mountain trails.
    D. Enjoying an at-home movie fest with a few friends.
    E. Flying to a foreign country.

4. When the weekend hits, you can be found:
    A. Enjoying a family event with the in-laws, spouse, kids, cat, and dog.
    B. Busy with your hobbies.
    C. Jogging through the neighborhood.
    D. On the couch, cuddled up with you-know-who.
    E. Attending an out-of-town social event.

5. A meal to you means, in one word:
   A. Fun.
   B. Wholesome.
   C. Quick.
   D. Healthy.
   E. Exciting.

Tally Up

Once you understand your cooking and eating styles, you can use the knowledge to select oils that are compatible with them. This, in turn, will enhance your olive oil experience. See how you scored below. I've made a few oil-wise choices for you to get started or to add to your current olive oil repertoire.

Mostly A's: The Extrovert.
Your Style: You are well-rounded, fun-loving, and people-oriented. You want an oil that is versatile and good for kids and animals. An all-purpose olive oil is ideal. An oil that will not be too exotic during family get-togethers is best.
Your Best Oils: Extra virgin olive oil, roasted garlic olive oil, and citrus olive oils.

Mostly B's. The Introvert.
Your Style: You are the intellectual, an independent individual who may live alone. You'd probably enjoy an olive oil that is good for you and versatile, as opposed to strong-flavored.
Your Best Oils: Extra virgin olive oil, basil olive oil, and citrus olive oils.

Mostly C's. The Outdoor Health Nut.
Your Style: You are a physical person, ready to hike in the summer, hit the gym in the winter. You're an active individual with a sense of adventure as long as it's healthful.
Your Best Oils: Light olive oil, extra virgin olive oil, and porcini olive oil.

Mostly D's. The Indoor Hermit.
Your Style: You are a sofa spud, with one hand on the remote con-

trol and the other in a bag of wholesome doggie treats. An afternoon of baking is up your alley.

Your Best Oils: Extra virgin olive oil and homemade flavored olive oils.

Mostly E's. The Adventurer.

Your Style: You are ready to travel for work or play. Trying new foods is what life is all about. You enjoy tasting new foods and flavors wherever you go, and "bland" is not in your vocabulary.

Your Best Oils: Pepper olive oil, porcini olive oil, rosemary olive oil, and oregano olive oil.

EPICUREAN ENJOYMENT

The common trait of people who travel to Europe to enjoy the world of olive oil is that they know why this liquid gold is priceless. By listening to and learning from each and every olive oil buff, I have collected the following tips—about the traditional Mediterranean-type diet and lifestyle—which I now pass along to you to give you a taste of Tuscany:

1. Eat breakfast, and use olive oil in your frying pan and muffin tin.
2. Enjoy lunch, and don't hesitate to use a vinegar-and-oil dressing on fresh greens . . .
3. . . . And to dip your French bread into olive oil.
4. Say yes to fish at least two to three times per week.
5. Say no to processed foods. Think fresh, organic, and natural.
6. Incorporate physical activity into your everyday lifestyle—for your heart and your soul's sakes.
7. Pamper yourself, your family, and your pets with olive oil and olive oil–based beauty products, naturally.
8. Try olive oil as your first line of action to treat health ailments before using a traditional medicine.
9. Learn to fine-tune your taste buds to enjoy natural foods, enhancing their flavors with Mother Nature's herbs and spices.
10. Chill and use olive oil and aromatic essential oils to de-stress and enjoy the wide world of olive oil mania.

The Golden Door Spa chefs, olive oil–smart John Deane, M.D., and Dr. Seth Roberts who turned to oil to maintain his weight, as well as the people at The Olive Press and the North American Olive Oil Association—and all the other unforgettable people in *The Healing Powers of Olive Oil*—get it. In their own individual ways, they understand that olive oil is an amazing folk medicine that is still embraced worldwide in the twenty-first century. You, like me and countless people around the world, can also reap the versatile benefits of olive oil without leaving home. Go ahead—enjoy the treasure that, after all these years, is still good as gold.

BEFORE YOU USE OLIVE OIL

You don't have to go to Spain, Italy, or Greece to enjoy the healing powers of olive oil. Whether you live on the West Coast, on the East Coast, in the Midwest, in the South, or in another country, you can find good local and imported olive oils that will bring you closer to achieving good health and well-being.

Keep in mind, however, that olive oil is not a magic bullet. Using it by itself or overindulging in the golden liquid to prevent or treat health ailments and lower your risk of disease isn't realistic.

Remember, the Mediterranean diet is more than just a diet. It is a lifestyle. By teaming meals based on vegetables, fruits, whole grains, fish, low-fat dairy products, and olive oil with daily physical activity, you can reap the healing benefits of the liquid gold and add years to your life.

When choosing an olive oil, remember to:

- Always check for the producing country's seal of authenticity— for instance, the COOC from California, the DOP from Italy, the AOC from France, the DOP from Greece, and the DO from Spain.
- Check the "use by" date.
- Check for winners of olive oil competitions. These olive oils will have seals, such as Gold, Silver, and Bronze medals, on their bottles.

Breakfast

In my twenties, I didn't believe in breakfast. But today, I can still hear my mom nag, "You should eat a bowl of cereal and a piece of fruit. It will give you energy for the day and keep you healthier as you grow up." It turns out Mom was right. So are all those breakfast-loving Europeans in the Mediterranean countries. Italians, Greeks, and Spaniards take time out for breakfast.

And these days, I do savor this meal, whether I'm at work or play at home, on a book tour, or out in the field doing research for a book. The fact is, breakfast is the most important meal of the day because it can rev up your metabolism and keep you burning calories all day long. This is key to staying lean and maintaining your ideal weight.

So, I have gotten into the habit of eating oatmeal, fruit, fresh orange juice, low-fat or nonfat yogurt, and coffee with low-fat milk. On special days (such as in a hotel room or on a Sunday morning at home), I do love special treats such as healthful muffins or pancakes. But, rather than turn to tasty treats that have a long list of ingredients that you can't pronounce, make your own scrumptious breakfast goodies. Here, take a look at some tasty, good-for-you recipes worth writing home to Mom about.

Blueberry Pancakes
Glorious Morning Muffins
Sweet Potato Biscuits
Tuscan Omelet

Blueberry Pancakes

1½ cups flour
¼ cup sugar
1 tablespoon baking powder
½ teaspoon baking soda
½ teaspoon salt

1¾ cups buttermilk
⅓ cup ricotta cheese
2 tablespoons Marsala Olive Oil
2 eggs
2 cups blueberries

In a mixing bowl, combine the dry ingredients. Make a well in the center and pour in buttermilk, ricotta, olive oil, and eggs. Stir just until the mixture is moistened. Fold in the blueberries. Lightly oil a griddle or large non-stick skillet over medium heat. Drop the batter by ¼ cups onto the hot griddle and spread gently into 4-inch rounds. Cook the pancakes 2–3 minutes. Turn the pancakes over and cook 1–2 more minutes. Repeat with the remaining batter. Place the pancakes on a cookie sheet and keep them warm in the oven while cooking the remaining batter. Serve them with blueberry sauce or pure maple syrup.

(*Source: Baking Sensational Sweets with California Olive Oil* by Gemma Sanita Sciabica)

Glorious Morning Muffins

❖ ❖ ❖

1½ cups organic unbleached all-purpose flour

½ cup organic granulated cane sugar

½ teaspoon baking soda

2 teaspoons cinnamon

½ teaspoon ground nutmeg

3 organic eggs or equivalent substitute

½ cup Spectrum Naturals Organic Canola Oil

¼ cup organic pure maple syrup

1 teaspoon organic pure vanilla extract

½ teaspoon sea salt

½ cup crushed or finely chopped pineapple, drained

¾ cup shredded organic carrots

¾ cup chopped almonds or walnuts

¼ cup shredded sweetened coconut

Spectrum Naturals Canola Spray Oil

Preheat the oven to 375°. In a large bowl, measure the flour, sugar, salt, baking soda, cinnamon, and nutmeg. Sift into another bowl. In a separate bowl, whisk together until well blended the eggs, Spectrum Naturals Organic Canola Oil, maple syrup, and vanilla. Stir in the drained pineapple. Pour this mixture all at once over the dry ingredients and mix lightly to combine. Stir in the carrots, almonds, and coconut. Spray a 12-cup muffin tin with Spectrum Naturals Canola Spray Oil. Spoon the batter evenly into the 12 cups, about 1/3 cup into each tin. Bake on the center rack of the preheated oven for about 22 minutes, until a cake tester inserted into the center of a muffin comes out clean.

Remove from the oven and turn out onto a platter. Cool to room temperature before storing in a covered container for up to two days. Makes 12 muffins.

Sweet Potato Biscuits

❖ ❖ ❖

1 cup unbleached flour
1 cup whole wheat pastry flour
1 tablespoon baking powder
½ teaspoon sea salt
Pinch cinnamon
⅓ cup Spectrum Naturals Organic
   Canola Oil

¾ cup peeled, cooked, and mashed
   sweet potato
2 teaspoons maple syrup
1–2 tablespoons milk

Pre-heat oven to 450°. Sift the dry ingredients together. Place the sifted dry ingredients into a food processor, add the oil, and blend. Blend the sweet potatoes into the mixture and add the maple syrup. Add the milk a small amount at a time until the dough begins to form into a ball. Process as little as possible. Place the dough ball on a lightly floured surface and knead lightly, 5 to 10 times. Roll it out to 3/4-inch thickness and cut it into rounds. Place the cut-out rounds on a lightly oiled cookie sheet and bake for about 12 minutes. Makes 12 biscuits.

Tuscan Omelet

❖ ❖ ❖

4 artichokes
1 lemon, cut in half
2 medium red potatoes
¾ cup thinly sliced crimini mushrooms or oak mushrooms
2 tablespoons thinly sliced fresh
   basil

4 plum tomatoes, seeded and
   finely diced
Olive and canola oil in a spray
   bottle or 2 teaspoons olive oil
4 eggs
8 egg whites
4 tablespoons grated Asiago cheese

Remove the stems and leaves from the artichokes and scoop out the feathery pulp that covers the hearts. Squeeze the juice of half a lemon over the hearts to prevent them from turning brown. Place the artichoke hearts into a pot of lightly salted water set over medium-high heat and bring to a simmer; simmer for 20 minutes, or until tender.

Meanwhile, place the potatoes into another pot of water set over medium-high heat and bring to a boil; boil for 20 minutes, or until the potatoes are tender and easily pierced by the tip of a sharp knife. Drain the potatoes, peel them, and cut them into small dices.

When the artichoke hearts are done, remove them from the water with a slotted spoon, dice finely, and transfer to a mixing bowl. Stir in the potatoes, mushrooms, basil, and tomatoes.

Spray or grease a non-stick pan with 1 teaspoon olive oil and set over medium heat. Add the artichoke-potato mixture; sauté, stirring, for 3–5 minutes, or until the mushrooms are soft. Remove from the heat and set aside.

Using an electric mixer or a fork, lightly beat the eggs and egg whites together until thoroughly blended. Set aside.

Spray or grease an 8-inch non-stick pan with olive oil and set over medium heat. Pour in 1/4 of the egg batter; cook for 2–3 minutes. Lift up the sides of the omelet to let the uncooked egg flow to the bottom of the pan. When the omelet is no longer liquid, scatter 1/4 of the cooked artichoke-potato mixture over the eggs; cook until the eggs are dry. If you wish, you can bake the omelet instead at 350° for 3–5 minutes to cook the eggs evenly.

Sprinkle the eggs with 1 tablespoon of Asiago cheese and gently fold the omelet in half with a rubber spatula; keep warm. Repeat the process to make 3 more omelets with the remaining eggs and artichoke-potato mixture. Serve immediately. Serves 4.

(Reprinted with permission from *The Golden Door Spa Cooks Light & Easy* by Chef Michel Stroot, published by Gibbs Smith, 2003)

Appetizers and Breads

An appetizer doesn't have to be fattening or unhealthy. Plenty of appetizers, such as these Mediterranean types, can include fresh vegetables, garlic, nuts, and olive oil. At Frantoio's Restaurant in Mill Valley, California, the menu includes an array of irresistible appetizers that each are fit for a meal by itself.

Not only will appetizers such as slices of warm homemade Olive Bread dipped in fresh extra virgin olive oil give you an Italian taste, they will curb your hunger pangs so you won't be tempted to overeat at lunch or dinner. And note, while dinner can be nutritious and delightful, to people who follow a true Mediterranean diet, it is the lightest meal of the day and eaten before 7:00 P.M. Appetizers like these can help you stay on track.

Artichoke Hearts Baked with Lemon and Romano Cheese
Olive Bread
Pan-Fried Japanese Eggplant in Chile Garlic Sauce
Vegetable Terrine Provençale

Artichoke Hearts Baked with Lemon and Romano Cheese

1 teaspoon finely grated lemon zest

1½ tablespoons fresh lemon juice, from about ½ lemon

3 tablespoons Spectrum Naturals Organic Greek Olive Oil

3 large cloves garlic, coarsely chopped

2 tablespoons chopped fresh mint leaves

Salt and pepper to taste

1 can artichoke hearts, drained and cut in half

6 sun-dried tomatoes, cut into thin slices

¼ cup grated Romano or soy Parmesan cheese

¼ cup fresh or store-bought plain bread crumbs

1 tablespoon Spectrum Naturals Daily Essential Flax Fiber

3 tablespoons coarsely chopped walnuts

Pre-heat the oven to 375°. In a small bowl, combine the lemon zest, lemon juice, olive oil, garlic, mint leaves, and salt and pepper to taste. Whisk to combine. Taste for seasonings. Spray a glass baking dish with Spectrum Naturals Olive Oil Spray. Arrange the halved artichoke hearts, cut side up, in a single layer in the prepared baking dish. Scatter the slices of sun-dried tomatoes evenly over the artichoke hearts. Into a small bowl, measure the grated cheese, bread crumbs, Spectrum Naturals Daily Essential Flax Fiber, and walnuts. Stir to combine. Spoon the lemon–olive oil mixture evenly over the artichoke hearts. Sprinkle the grated cheese–bread crumb mixture evenly over the top. Bake for 20–25 minutes, until the artichoke hearts are heated through and the topping is golden brown. Serves 4.

(Recipe created by Claire Criscuolo, restaurateur)

Olive Bread

❖ ❖ ❖

2½ teaspoons active dry yeast
4 cups unbleached all-purpose
  flour
⅓ cup white wine
⅓ cup pureed Kalamata or other
  brine-cured black olives (about
  30 olives)

3 tablespoons olive oil (preferably
  extra virgin)
¾ teaspoon salt
¼ teaspoon white pepper

In a small bowl, proof the yeast in ½ cup lukewarm water with ½ cup flour for 30 minutes. In a bowl, combine the wine, olive puree, oil, salt, white pepper, and ¼ cup water. Stir in the yeast mixture and 2–2½ cups flour, and combine the dough well. Knead the dough on a well-floured surface for 15 minutes, incorporating more flour as necessary to keep it from sticking. Put the dough in a well-buttered bowl, turn it to coat it with the butter, and let it rise, covered with plastic wrap, in a warm place for 1 hour, or until it has doubled in bulk. Punch down the dough, form it into an oval about 8 inches long, and put it on a well-buttered baking sheet. Score the top of the bread diagonally with a sharp knife at 1-inch intervals and let the bread rise in warm place for 30–40 minutes, or until it has almost doubled in bulk. Bake the bread in a pre-heated 375° oven for 35–45 minutes, or until it is golden and sounds hollow when tapped. Transfer it to a rack and let it cool. Makes 1 loaf.

(*Source:* www.epicurean.com)

Pan-Fried Japanese Eggplant in Chile Garlic Sauce

❖ ❖ ❖

SAUCE
2 tablespoons orange juice
1 tablespoon low-sodium soy
  sauce
1 tablespoon sugar

1 teaspoon Thai chile sauce
1 teaspoon orange zest
½ teaspoon sea salt

¼ cup Spectrum Naturals High-
  Heat Canola Oil
1 pound Japanese eggplant, cut
  into 1-inch cubes

3 cloves garlic, minced
1 tablespoon minced ginger

Stir together the sauce ingredients and set aside. Heat the oil over high heat and add the eggplant to the pan. Cook, stirring frequently, for 5-6 minutes, until golden brown on all sides. Lower the heat to medium and transfer the browned eggplant to a plate lined with paper toweling. Add the garlic and ginger to the pan and cook, stirring constantly, for 30 seconds. Pour the orange juice mixture into the pan and bring it to a boil. Reduce the heat to medium and let the juice mixture boil until it has reduced to a syrupy consistency. Add the eggplant back to the pan and toss it to coat. Cook the eggplant until heated through, and serve. Serves 4.

Vegetable Terrine Provençale

❖ ❖ ❖

2 medium eggplants, peeled and
   sliced lengthwise into ½-inch
   strips
3 large zucchini, cut lengthwise
   into ½-inch strips
Olive oil and canola oil in a spray
   bottle or 2 tablespoons plus 2
   teaspoons olive oil
¼ cup balsamic vinegar
½ teaspoon kosher salt, optional
1 teaspoon freshly ground black
   pepper, optional

3 medium red bell peppers
2 ounces thinly sliced smoked
   salmon
¾ cup part-skim ricotta cheese
20 fresh basil leaves, cut into very
   thin strips
Mixed greens for serving, washed
   and patted dry
Rosemary sprigs for garnish
Kalamata or Niçoise olives for garnish

Lightly spray the eggplant and zucchini with 1 teaspoon olive oil and transfer to a large mixing bowl. Stir in the balsamic vinegar, salt, and black pepper, if using; marinate 30 minutes.

Pre-heat a grill, stovetop grill, or broiler. Lightly spray or brush the red bell peppers with 1 teaspoon olive oil; grill or broil for 5 minutes, turning so that all sides are charred. Transfer to a plastic bag and seal; set aside for about 10 minutes, or until the peppers are cool enough to handle. Remove the skin and seeds, and cut each into 10 equal-size pieces. Set aside.

Remove the eggplant from the marinade and spray or brush with 1 teaspoon olive oil, if necessary. Grill or broil 3–4 minutes per side, or until the eggplant just begins to soften. Remove from the grill and set aside. Remove the zucchini from the marinade; grill or broil 3–4 minutes per side, or until it begins to soften.

Line a 9½-x-2½-inch terrine pan with plastic wrap, and spray or brush with 1 teaspoon olive oil. Place the smoked salmon into the pan, arranging it so that the bottom of the pan is covered. Place 4 slices of grilled eggplant on top of the salmon. Mist the eggplant with 1 tea-spoon olive oil. Using a spatula, spread on a layer of ricotta cheese. Scatter some of the basil strips on top of the cheese. Press on 5 to 6 grilled zucchini slices, mist with 1 teaspoon olive oil, and spread with another layer of ricotta and basil. Add a layer of roasted red pepper and mist again with 1 teaspoon olive oil. Top with another layer of ricotta and basil. Repeat the process until all the grilled vegetables have been used, finishing with a layer of zucchini and eggplant and a final misting of olive oil. Gently press down, and cover the terrine with plastic wrap. Press the terrine with another empty terrine pan or loaf pan of the same size; refrigerate overnight.

Carefully remove the vegetable terrine from the pan by pulling up on the plastic wrap. Place on a cutting board. Using a sharp knife, carefully cut it into 1-inch slices. Place the terrine slices on a bed of mixed greens and garnish with rosemary sprigs and olives; serve. The Vegetable Terrine Provençale can be kept in the refrigerator, covered, for three to four days.

(Reprinted with permission from *The Golden Door Spa Cooks Light & Easy* by Chef Michel Stroot, published by Gibbs Smith, 2003)

Salads

Salads can be a great weapon in the battle against the bulge, but here's something you might not have heard: wholesome salads can be slimming as well as beautifying and antiaging when they supply just the right nutrients.

To me, a salad often is a meal by itself. A salad should be chock-full of fresh vegetables, and fish is also an excellent ingredient. To enhance a salad and make a delicious treat, top it off with olive oil. No matter what type of olive oil you choose, you can create a wonderful slimming salad that is a complete meal or to-die-for side dish for just you or for an elegant dinner party.

These meal-sized salads are packed with all kinds of tasty, nutrient-rich ingredients, such as juicy tomatoes, flavorful feta cheese, and even black olives. Add garlic, onion, spices, and vinegar—which many of these salads contain—and you've got a heart-healthy, hearty, nutritious dish to eat solo or to share with guests for lunch or dinner.

Golden Door Salad with Tonnata Dressing
Greek Salad
Panzanella (Tuscan Bread and Tomato Salad)
Spring Wild Rice Salad

Golden Door Salad with Tonnata Dressing

DRESSING

Olive oil and canola oil in a spray
  bottle or 1 teaspoon olive oil
½ medium onion, finely diced
1 tablespoon minced garlic
3 anchovy fillets, rinsed and patted dry
½ cup silken tofu (about 5 ounces)
½ cup water
2 tablespoons fresh lemon juice

1 teaspoon fresh thyme leaves or ½
  teaspoon dried thyme
3 ounces canned light tuna packed
  in water, drained
½ teaspoon freshly ground black
  pepper
⅓ cup chopped parsley
2 tablespoons capers, drained

SALAD

1 cup French-style green beans	4 cups baby romaine lettuce,
4 small red potatoes	washed and patted dry
Olive oil and canola oil in a spray	2 red tomatoes, cut into wedges
bottle or 1 teaspoon olive oil	2 yellow tomatoes, cut into wedges
2 eggs, hard-cooked	8 ounces canned light tuna packed
	in water, drained

To prepare the dressing, spray or grease a non-stick pan with olive oil and set over medium heat. Add the onion and garlic; sauté, stirring, for 3–5 minutes, or until the onion is translucent and soft. Transfer the mixture to a blender or food processor fitted with a metal blade. Add the anchovies, silken tofu, water, lemon juice, thyme, and tuna; process until smooth. Add the black pepper, parsley, and capers; pulse to incorporate. Refrigerate until ready to serve. Makes 1 cup.

To prepare the salad, bring a large pot of water to a boil and prepare a bowl of ice water. Immerse the green beans in the boiling water for 4–5 minutes, or until the beans are tender. Drain the beans and plunge them into the ice water for 30 seconds to stop the cooking process. Drain.

Place the potatoes into a small pot, add enough water to cover, set the pot over medium-high heat, and bring to a simmer. Simmer for 20 minutes, or until the potatoes are just tender. (Be careful not to overcook them or they will fall apart when you try to slice them.) When the potatoes are done, drain them in a colander and run under cold water to stop the cooking process. Drain. Slice the cooled potatoes and spray or brush with olive oil. Set aside.

Peel the hard-cooked eggs, remove and discard the yolks, and chop the egg whites finely.

Place equal portions of the romaine leaves on chilled salad plates. Arrange the potato slices, red and yellow tomato wedges, and blanched green beans around the lettuce. Place equal portions of tuna on each plate and sprinkle each with chopped egg whites. Drizzle each salad with 2 tablespoons Tonnata Dressing. Tonnata Dressing can be kept in the refrigerator, covered, for up to 5 days.

(Reprinted with permission from *The Golden Door Spa Cooks Light & Easy* by Chef Michel Stroot, published by Gibbs Smith, 2003)

Greek Salad

❖ ❖ ❖

DRESSING
½ cup olive oil
1 clove garlic, minced
4 teaspoons sugar
¼ teaspoon salt

⅓ cup red wine vinegar
2 teaspoons minced parsley
½ teaspoon basil
¼ teaspoon pepper

SALAD
Tomatoes
Cucumbers
Red onions

Black olives
½ cup crumbled feta cheese

Mix the dressing and set aside. Chop the veggies, add the crumbled feta, and toss with the dressing. Serve immediately, or refrigerate to marinate several hours or overnight.

(*Source:* Spectrum Naturals)

Panzanella
(Tuscan Tomato and Bread Salad)

❖ ❖ ❖

4–5 large vine-ripened tomatoes,
   cut into large cubes or wedges
½ pound stale country-style
   Italian bread, crusts removed
   and cubed (about 8 cups)
1¼ cups thinly sliced red onions
2 teaspoons minced garlic
¼ cup The Olive Press
   Champagene Balsamic Vinegar

½ cup The Olive Press Extra
   Virgin Olive Oil
1 bunch fresh basil, stems
   removed, washed and spun dry,
   torn into pieces
Sea salt and freshly ground black
   pepper

In a large bowl, combine the tomatoes, bread, and onions. In a small bowl, whisk together the garlic, vinegar, and olive oil. Pour the dressing over the bread salad and let sit for 30 minutes at room temperature. Add the basil and salt and pepper to taste, and toss to combine. Serves 4–6.

(*Source:* The Olive Press)

Spring Wild Rice Salad

❖ ❖ ❖

½ cup wild rice, rinsed
2½ cups water
1 bay leaf
¼ cup fresh lemon juice
1 tablespoon olive oil
1 cup corn kernels
½ cup chopped scallions
2 large plum tomatoes, seeded and
diced

½ cup finely chopped parsley
2 teaspoons finely chopped fresh
lemon thyme or common thyme
1 teaspoon kosher salt, optional
Freshly ground black pepper to
taste, optional

Combine the rice, water, and bay leaf in a small pot set over medium-high heat; cover and bring to a simmer. Simmer for 35 minutes, or until the rice is tender. Transfer to a mixing bowl and let cool. Remove the bay leaf. Stir in the lemon juice, olive oil, corn, scallions, tomatoes, parsley, thyme, and salt, if using. Mix well and refrigerate for 30 minutes. Season with black pepper, if desired.

Note: Freshly squeezed lemon juice and lemon thyme give this salad a bright, tangy taste. Serve it at room temperature for the best flavor. If you can't find lemon thyme, use the more common variety.

(Reprinted with permission from *The Golden Door Spa Cooks Light & Easy* by Chef Michel Stroot, published by Gibbs Smith, 2003.)

Vegetables and Vegetarian Dishes

At 18, I became a vegan. I admit this announcement did not make my mother happy. She made superb dishes—all types of cuisine—from breaded veal to beef stew from scratch. After all, as a child of the fifties, I grew up on meat and potatoes. But my mom visited Europe when I was 10, and when she came back home, our meals were often more creative and daring. Think snails and squid.

I don't know if it was nutritionist Adelle Davis or the popularity of health food stores that influenced me. Perhaps it was both. I do know, however, that eating fresh vegetables, fruits, grains, yogurt, and nuts has worked to keep me—a 5-foot 5-inch woman—at 122 pounds and size 4–6 for decades.

During the gathering of these Mediterranean recipes, I learned that I can make my diet much tastier and more healthful by adding fresh onions, garlic, spices, and olive oil—especially flavored oils. The European flair is exciting to enjoy at home, especially if you can't whisk off to Italy, Spain, or Greece.

Sesame-Almond Vegetable Sauté
Shallot-Herb Stuffed Potatoes
Mashed Sweet Potatoes
Summer Vegetable and Organic Tofu Tacos

Sesame-Almond Vegetable Sauté

½ small (about 2 pounds) butternut or buttercup squash, peeled, seeded, and cut into ¾-inch pieces (2 cups)
1 cup baby carrots
⅓ cup chicken broth or water
1½ cups cauliflower florets (about 1½ inches long)
2 cups broccoli florets (about 1½ inches long)

⅓ cup slivered almonds
¼ cup extra virgin olive oil
1 medium onion, cut into thin wedges
1 clove garlic, minced
2–3 teaspoons fresh thyme leaves
½ teaspoon salt
¼ teaspoon red pepper flakes
1 tablespoon toasted sesame seeds

In a Dutch oven or large skillet, combine the squash, carrots, and chicken broth. Cook over medium-high heat until the broth is steaming. Cover and cook 3 minutes. Add the cauliflower and broccoli; cover and cook 2–3 minutes longer, or just until the squash is tender and the broccoli is brightened. Drain and set aside.

In a small skillet over medium-high heat, cook the almonds 5–7 minutes, or until lightly golden brown, stirring frequently. Remove from the heat.

In a very large skillet or Dutch oven, heat the olive oil over medium heat. Add the onion and garlic; cook and stir 2–3 minutes, or until the onion is softened. Increase the heat to medium-high. Add the well-drained vegetable mixture, thyme, salt, and red pepper flakes. Cook and stir until hot and tender. Stir in the almonds and turn into a serving dish. Sprinkle with the sesame seeds. Serves 12.

(*Source:* North American Olive Oil Association)

Shallot-Herb Stuffed Potatoes

❖ ❖ ❖

4 medium potatoes
1 teaspoon canola oil
2 teaspoons olive oil
1¼ cups sliced shallots
2 teaspoons fresh thyme leaves
1 teaspoon freshly ground black pepper
1 tablespoon balsamic vinegar

¼ cup Vegetable Broth (recipe below)
½ cup low-fat cottage cheese
1 tablespoon whole-grain mustard
2 tablespoons grated Parmesan or Asiago cheese
2 tablespoons chopped fresh parsley

VEGETABLE BROTH

1 medium leek, sliced and washed well
2 celery ribs, coarsely chopped
1 large carrot, coarsely chopped
1 medium onion, coarsely chopped
3 large cabbage leaves
5 cloves garlic
4 sprigs fresh parsley

2 sprigs fresh basil
2 sprigs fresh thyme
1 bay leaf
1 teaspoon kosher salt, optional
1 teaspoon freshly ground black pepper
1 quart water

To make the Vegetable Broth, combine all ingredients in a large stockpot. Set the pot over medium-high heat and bring to a boil. Reduce the heat to medium-low and simmer, uncovered, for 1 hour, or until the liquid has reduced in volume by about a third.

Using a fine-mesh sieve or colander lined with cheesecloth, strain into a large bowl or other container. Press gently on solids to remove all the liquid; discard the solids. Use immediately, or refrigerate or freeze for later use. Vegetable Broth can be kept in the refrigerator, covered, for three to four days or in the freezer for up to one month.

To make the stuffed potatoes, pre-heat the oven to 375°. Brush the potatoes with canola oil and place on a baking sheet. Bake the potatoes for 1 hour, or until fork-tender. Remove from the oven; set aside until they are just cool enough to handle.

Meanwhile, heat the olive oil in non-stick pan over medium-high heat. Add the shallots; sauté, stirring, for about 5 minutes, or until golden brown. Stir in the thyme and black pepper; cook for another 2 minutes. Deglaze the pan by adding the balsamic vinegar and broth, stirring with a wooden spoon to loosen any flavorful browned bits. Reduce the heat to medium; simmer for 2–3 minutes. Set aside.

When the potatoes are cool enough to handle but still warm, cut a thin layer off the top of each (holding it horizontally, as you would serve a baked potato); scoop out the flesh, leaving a ½-inch-thick shell.

Combine the scooped-out potato, cottage cheese, mustard, and caramelized shallots in a mixing bowl; mix well with a spatula. Spoon the mixture back into the potato shells, mounding it so that the potatoes are well-rounded. Sprinkle with the grated cheese; return the stuffed potatoes and their tops to the oven for 15 minutes, or until the cheese is golden brown and the tops are crispy. Place a potato on each warmed plate, prop the top at a diagonal so that the stuffing can be seen, sprinkle with parsley, and serve immediately.

(Reprinted with permission from *The Golden Door Spa Cooks Light & Easy* by Chef Michel Stroot, published by Gibbs Smith, 2003)

Mashed Sweet Potatoes

❖ ❖ ❖

4 large sweet potatoes (about 5 pounds), peeled and quartered

Extra light olive oil for greasing casserole

¼ cup extra light olive oil

1 medium onion, chopped

2–3 teaspoons grated fresh ginger-root

¼ cup pure maple syrup

1 egg

2 tablespoons grated orange peel (about 2 oranges)

1 teaspoon cinnamon

1 teaspoon salt

½ teaspoon cardamom, optional

⅛ teaspoon cayenne pepper

2 slices cinnamon bread, torn into 1-inch pieces

2 teaspoons extra light olive oil

Place the potatoes in a Dutch oven with enough water to cover. Bring to a boil. Reduce the heat to medium-low, cover loosely, and simmer 15–25 minutes or until tender.* Drain well in a colander, place in a large bowl, and set aside.

Heat oven to 350°. Lightly oil a 2-quart casserole with olive oil. In a medium skillet or saucepan, heat the ¼-cup olive oil over medium heat. Add the onion and gingerroot; cook and stir until tender.

Lightly mash the potatoes with a spoon or potato masher. Add the onion mixture and remaining ingredients except for the cinnamon bread and 2 teaspoons olive oil. For a smoother consistency, beat with a mixer to blend. For a chunkier mixture, mash with a potato masher or wooden spoon to blend. Spoon into the prepared casserole.

In a food processor or blender, process the bread pieces until completely chopped. Blend in the remaining 2 teaspoons of olive oil. Sprinkle over the potato mixture. Bake 35–45 minutes, or until lightly browned and thoroughly hot. Serves 18–20.

(*Source:* North American Olive Oil Association)

---

* Potatoes are tender when a knife can easily be inserted into the thickest parts with little or no resistance. For a smoother casserole, cook the potatoes until very tender. For a slightly chunkier casserole, cook the potatoes just until the knife can be inserted.

Summer Vegetable and Organic Tofu Tacos

❖ ❖ ❖

2 teaspoons Spectrum Naturals
  Organic California Extra
  Virgin Olive Oil
1 medium sweet onion, coarsely
  chopped
5 cloves garlic, coarsely chopped
2 large ripe tomatoes, coarsely
  chopped (include juices)
1 small carrot, thinly sliced
2 medium green bell peppers,
  seeded and coarsely chopped
2 teaspoons dried oregano
2 teaspoons cumin
1 teaspoon chipotle powder
14 ounces extra firm organic tofu,
  drained and crumbled

2 tablespoons sliced almonds
1 medium zucchini, small cubes
Salt and pepper to taste
1 tablespoon Spectrum Naturals
  Organic Toasted Pumpkin Seed
  Oil
¼ cup chopped fresh cilantro
2 tablespoons freshly squeezed
  lime juice (about ½ lime)
1 tablespoon Spectrum Naturals
  Organic Flaxseed Oil
12 crisp corn taco shells, trans
  fat–free
1 cup Avocado Cream

AVOCADO CREAM

2 medium cloves garlic
1 jalapeño pepper, stem removed
2 tablespoons pumpkin seeds
¼ cup coarsely chopped fresh
  cilantro

1 ripe avocado
½ cup organic plain low-fat yogurt
2 teaspoons Spectrum Naturals
  Organic Flaxseed Oil
Salt to taste

Heat the olive oil in a large skillet over medium heat. Add the onion, garlic, tomatoes, carrot, bell peppers, oregano, cumin, chipotle powder, crumbled tofu, almonds, and zucchini. Sprinkle with the salt and pepper. Using a wooden spoon, turn the ingredients to coat them with the oil. Cook 8–10 minutes, stirring occasionally, until the peppers are crisp-tender.

Add the toasted pumpkin seed oil, cilantro, and lime juice. Stir well to combine. Cook for a minute to heat through. Remove from the heat and stir in the flaxseed oil. Taste for seasonings. When ready to serve, spoon about ½ cup into each taco shell. Top with a heaping tablespoon of Avocado Cream. Serves 6.

AVOCADO CREAM

Place the garlic cloves, stemmed jalapeño pepper, pumpkin seeds, and cilantro into a food processor fitted with a metal blade. Cover and process for about 10 seconds to mince. Cut the avocado in half, remove the pit, and scoop the flesh out into the processor bowl. Add the yogurt, flaxseed oil, and salt. Cover and process for about 10 seconds, until blended and smooth. Taste for seasonings. Makes 1 cup.

Pasta

Hot pasta paired with fresh herbs and fresh French bread dipped in warm olive oil are popular combinations in the Mediterranean diet. Pasta with an assortment of vegetables, fish, garlic, onions, and olive oil is not only a scrumptious delight, but it is a healthful meal.

Think whole wheat pasta (its fiber content is higher). It's low in fat and sodium, and has 180 calories per ¾ cup. Also, while this type of pasta is whole grain and has no preservatives, it's also free of trans fat and cholesterol. Plus, it contains iron, riboflavin, folic acid, thiamin, and niacin. What's more, I have learned to ignore store-bought pasta sauce (its sodium content is off the charts) and replace it with fresh tomatoes. (I did find one that contains olive oil and boasts of less sodium.)

One nutritionist zapped sodium from his daily diet to lower his blood-pressure numbers. He told me that he makes his own low-sodium sauce with potassium-rich tomato paste—which makes sense, especially if you whip up a large batch and freeze it in several containers. If you, too, switch to whole wheat pasta and fresh vegetables, and add olive oil and homemade tomato paste–based sauces to your pastas, you'll come closer to a traditional Mediterranean diet, which can lead you on the path to better heart health and a longer life.

P.S.: Join me and toss out that butter or margarine that were popular back in the 1950s and '60s. You can learn to dip your bread in olive oil—a European custom that is practiced in Italian restaurants from Lake Tahoe to Tuscany and in homes around the world.

Pasta E' Piselli
Quick Two-Tomato Sauce with Black Olives
Angel Hair Pasta with Diced Tomatoes, Edamame Beans, Basil
and Virgin Olive Oil
Asparagus and Wild Mushroom Pappardelle

Pasta E' Piselli

❖ ❖ ❖

1 pound tubetti pasta or other
   short tube pasta
3 tablespoons Spectrum Naturals
   Organic Spanish Extra Virgin
   Olive Oil
1 large sweet onion, coarsely
   chopped
6 large cloves garlic, sliced
1 pint sweet grape tomatoes
¼ cup chopped fresh basil leaves
   or 1 teaspoon dried
1 teaspoon dried oregano

Salt
Pepper to taste
10-ounce box frozen green peas
2 cups reserved cooking water from
   pasta
1 tablespoon Spectrum Naturals
   Organic Flaxseed Oil with
   Lemon
3 tablespoons freshly grated
   Pecorino cheese
Romano cheese, optional

Bring a large pot of lightly salted water to a boil over high heat. Add the pasta and cook according to the package directions. Before draining the pasta, reserve 2 cups of the cooking water. (A good way to remember to reserve the water is to set a measuring cup into your colander as a reminder.) After draining the pasta, transfer it to a serving bowl.

Meanwhile, heat the olive oil in a large, deep skillet over medium heat. Add the onion, garlic, grape tomatoes, basil, and oregano. Sprinkle with the salt and pepper, then stir to coat. Cover and cook for about 15 minutes, stirring occasionally, until the tomatoes are soft and the sauce looks creamy. Add the peas and reserved cooking water. Stir to combine. Cover and continue cooking for about 5 minutes, stirring occasionally, until the peas are heated through and the sauce has reduced slightly. Taste for seasonings. Pour the sauce over the cooked pasta, using a rubber spatula to scrape any juices from the skillet. Using two wooden spoons, toss to combine. Taste for seasonings. Drizzle the Spectrum Naturals Organic Flaxseed Oil with Lemon evenly over the pasta. Top with additional black pepper and grated cheese if desired.

Serves 4–6.

Quick Two-Tomato Sauce with Black Olives

❖ ❖ ❖

2 tablespoons Spectrum Naturals Organic Canola Oil

1 medium yellow onion, minced

4 cloves garlic, minced

4 cups canned diced tomatoes or peeled, seeded, and diced ripe garden tomatoes

⅓ cup chopped dried tomatoes

⅓ cup Niçoise or black olives, pitted

3 tablespoons chopped fresh parsley

3 tablespoons chopped fresh basil

3 tablespoons Spectrum Naturals Cold-Pressed Extra Virgin Olive Oil

2 tablespoons Spectrum Naturals Organic Red Wine Vinegar

Salt

Freshly ground pepper

Warm the canola oil in a 2- or 3-quart saucepan over medium heat. Add the onions and sauté for 5 minutes. Add the garlic, diced tomatoes, and dried tomatoes. Simmer for 15 minutes. Add the olives and continue to simmer until all of the juice from the tomatoes has evaporated. Stir in the parsley and basil. Simmer for 5 more minutes. Stir in the olive oil and vinegar. Simmer for 5 more minutes, stirring often. Season with salt and freshly ground pepper. Serve over pasta, as an accompaniment to grilled or steamed fish, or simply spread cold on toast rounds as an appetizer. Makes about 2½ cups.

Angel Hair Pasta with Diced Tomatoes, Edamame Beans, Basil, and Virgin Olive Oil

❖ ❖ ❖

8 ounces soy angel hair pasta
1 cup edamame beans
Olive oil and canola oil in a spray
   bottle or 1 teaspoon olive oil
2 teaspoons minced garlic
4 vine-ripened tomatoes, seeded
   and finely diced

2 tablespoons extra virgin olive oil
⅓ cup thinly sliced fresh basil
6 tablespoons grated Asiago or imported Pecorino cheese
4 fresh basil leaves for garnish

Boil a large pot of water and add the pasta, stirring it once with a fork to prevent sticking. Cook for 8–10 minutes, or until al dente. Transfer to a colander, drain, and set aside.

Meanwhile, bring a small pot of water to a simmer over medium-high heat. Add the edamame beans; cook for 3–4 minutes. The beans should still be firm and a vivid green color. Drain and set aside.

Spray or grease a skillet with 1 teaspoon olive oil and set over medium heat. Add the garlic; stir for 1–2 minutes, or until softened. Add the tomatoes; cook for 1 minute, just to heat through. Add the cooked pasta, edamame beans, and 2 tablespoons extra virgin olive oil; cook, tossing, for 2–3 minutes longer, to heat through. Stir in the basil.

Place equal portions of the hot pasta into warm bowls and sprinkle each with cheese. Garnish with a basil leaf and serve.

(Reprinted with permission from *The Golden Door Spa Cooks Light & Easy* by Chef Michel Stroot, published by Gibbs Smith, 2003)

Asparagus and Wild Mushroom Pappardelle

❖ ❖ ❖

8–12 ounces fresh pappardelle
  pasta*
3 tablespoons The Olive Press
  Arbequina extra virgin olive oil
½ bunch asparagus, cut into 1-
  inch lengths
½ large onion, halved and sliced
¼ pound wild or cultivated mushrooms, cleaned and cut into
  bite-sized pieces

Salt and freshly ground pepper to
  taste
¾ cup dry white wine
2 tomatoes, chopped
2 tablespoons chopped Italian
  parsley
2 tablespoons freshly grated
  Parmesan cheese
The Olive Press Arbequina extra
virgin olive oil, to drizzle

Bring a large pot of salted water to a boil for the pasta. Begin cooking the pasta about 5 minutes before the sauce is ready.

Pre-heat a large sauté pan. Add the 3 tablespoons olive oil and then the asparagus. Cook approximately 1 minute. Add the onion and mushrooms, and cook an additional minute. Season with salt and pepper. Deglaze with the wine and continue cooking until reduced by half, about 5 minutes. Remove from the heat and stir in the chopped tomatoes.

Drain the cooked pasta and add it to the sauce. Add the parsley and toss lightly. Check the seasonings and adjust as needed.

Divide the pasta among 4 serving bowls, top with the Parmesan, and drizzle with extra virgin olive oil. Serves 4.

(*Source:* The Olive Press)

*Fresh pappardelle is available packaged and freshly cut in upscale markets and specialty pasta shops.

Poultry

Poultry, such as chicken and turkey, is included in the traditional Mediterranean Diet pyramid. These days, on rare occasions, I will celebrate a holiday such as Thanskgiving and purchase an organic turkey. There are healthful benefits (lean cuts of poultry boasts protein and can fill you up, not out) to having a bird in the house. And, of course, if you have a cat and two bird dogs, they will be in heaven. (No bones to the pets, please.)

Not only can you cook it up with fresh herbs, onion, and olive oil, but you can make a healthful turkey soup. I did just that last Thanksgiving and was truly thankful. I had soup to freeze, and each time I took out a container of it, I could add plenty of fresh vegetables (and olive oil) to flavor it, with no worries about the high sodium content found in store-bought soups.

Balsamic-Braised Chicken Thighs
Seared Boneless Breast of Chicken Stuffed with Spinach and Basil
Herbed Roast Turkey

Balsamic-Braised Chicken Thighs

2 pounds boneless, skinless
   chicken thighs
¼ teaspoon organic sea salt
¼ teaspoon freshly ground pepper
2 tablespoons Spectrum Naturals
   Organic Extra Virgin Olive Oil
1 cup diced onion

¾ cup Spectrum Naturals Organic
   Balsamic Vinegar
1 teaspoon minced fresh thyme
1 bay leaf
½ cup organic chicken stock
2 tablespoons organic honey

Season the chicken thighs with the salt and pepper. Heat a large skillet over medium-high heat. When hot, swirl with the 2 tablespoons olive oil, and brown the chicken on all sides. Remove the chicken to a plate, and sauté the onions until deeply bronzed.

Deglaze the pan with ¼ cup balsamic vinegar. Stir in the minced thyme, ground pepper, bay leaf, remaining ½ cup balsamic vinegar, chicken stock, and honey. Bring to a boil and return the thighs to the pan. Reduce the heat to low, cover, and simmer vigorously for 20–30 minutes, turning several times, until the chicken is cooked through and the sauce has become concentrated. Serve with roasted carrots. Serves 6.

Seared Boneless Breast of Chicken Stuffed with Spinach and Basil

❖ ❖ ❖

4 boneless chicken breasts
4 tablespoons Spectrum Naturals
  Super Canola Oil
4 cloves garlic, finely minced
24 spinach leaves, very coarsely
  chopped

16 large basil leaves
Salt and ground pepper
4 tablespoons Spectrum Naturals
  Spread

Lay the chicken breasts flat on your work surface. With a very sharp knife, create a pocket by cutting an incision horizontally through the middle of each breast, leaving the breast completely attached on one side. Heat a non-stick pan over low heat and add 2 tablespoons of the Spectrum Naturals Super Canola Oil. Add the garlic and simmer for 1 minute, then add the spinach and basil, and cook until just wilted, about 45 seconds. Season with the salt and pepper, and allow to cool. Combine the Spectrum Naturals Spread and cooled spinach mixture. Stuff the chicken breasts with equal parts of this mixture. Wipe the non-stick pan clean, place it over moderate heat, and add the remaining Super Canola Oil. Add the breasts and cook for approximately 4–5 minutes on each side, or until the chicken is cooked and the spinach is heated through. Remove the chicken from the pan and allow to rest for 3–5 minutes. Serves 4.

(Recipe created by Chef Gary Jenanyan)

Herbed Roast Turkey

❖ ❖ ❖

16–18-pound turkey, thawed if frozen
1 medium onion, cut into wedges
2 ribs celery, cut into 2-inch pieces
2 medium carrots, cut into 2-inch pieces
4–5 stems each of fresh sage, rosemary, and thyme, if desired

3 cloves garlic
⅓ cup chopped fresh sage leaves
¼ cup fresh rosemary leaves
3 tablespoons fresh thyme leaves
½ teaspoon salt
½ teaspoon pepper
⅓ plus ½ cup virgin olive oil

Heat oven to 325°. Remove the giblets and neck from the turkey; discard or save for broth, if desired. Rinse the cavity of the turkey and pat dry. Sprinkle the inside of the turkey with salt and pepper. Place the onion, celery, carrot, and, if desired, 1–2 stems each of the sage, rosemary, and thyme inside the turkey. Place the turkey on a rack in a roasting pan; set aside.

In a food processor or blender, chop the garlic until fine. Add the herb leaves; pulse until coarsely chopped. Add the salt and pepper. With the machine running, add the ⅓ cup olive oil and process until well blended.

Carefully separate (but do not remove) the skin from the meat on the breast of the turkey. Rub 2 tablespoons of the herb mixture between the meat and skin. Replace the skin. If desired, add 1 cup water or broth to the pan under the rack. Roast the turkey 1 hour.

Meanwhile, blend the remaining ½ cup olive oil into the remaining herb mixture. If desired, bundle the remaining herb stems together to form a "basting brush." After 1 hour of roasting, baste the turkey with part of the herb mixture.

Continue roasting the turkey 2½–3¼ hours* or until the internal temperature of the thickest part of the thigh is 170° and the juice runs clear, basting every hour. If necessary, cover the breast of the turkey with foil to prevent over-browning during roasting. Remove from oven and let stand 10–15 minutes before carving. Serves 16–20.

(*Source:* North American Olive Oil Association)

---

*The total roasting time will be about 12–20 minutes per pound, depending on the size of the turkey. Check the turkey wrapper for additional timing information. This olive oil–herb mixture can also be used when roasting only a turkey breast, and is also excellent on roasted or grilled chicken or pork.

Fish

While I prefer to be a strict vegetarian, it's a challenge to do it right and maintain good health. I know that I need essential fatty acids for good health. So, two to three times per week, I try to include fresh salmon or tuna in my diet. In my early teens, I do recall indulging in lobster, trout, halibut, shrimp, and scallops.

I recall a meal at Cannery Row in Monterey, California. It was the first time that I had the Cioppino experience—fun, and it is for the uninhibited fish lover. Mediterranean people do eat and love fresh, grilled fish. And, fish does play a role in the health perks of Mediterranean diets.

Cioppino
Halibut with Caper Sauce
Simple Salmon

Cioppino

¼ cup Marsala Olive Fruit Oil
1 onion, diced
6 cloves garlic, chopped
1 bell pepper, diced
¾ cup wine
4 cups chopped fresh or canned
    tomatoes
4 tablespoons tomato paste
Salt, pepper, and red hot pepper
    flakes to taste
2 bay leaves (remove before serving)

½ cup chopped fresh basil and/or
    parsley
½ pound cod, cut into 2-inch
    cubes
1 pound crab (Alaskan King,
    thawed)
1 pound shrimp
2 dozen clams or mussels
½ pound scallops

In a Dutch oven, add the oil, onions, garlic, and bell pepper. Cook over medium heat until soft. Add the wine and cook 1 minute. Add the tomatoes, tomato paste, salt, pepper, red hot pepper flakes, and bay leaves. Simmer for 15 minutes, covered, then add the basil. Add the cod and cook for about 5 minutes. Add the remaining fish and cook, covered, for 5 minutes, or until the clams open. Discard any unopened clams. Serve in soup bowls with toasted crusty Italian bread slices.*

VARIATIONS
Flounder fillets or lobster, cubed
2 cups small potatoes, cubed
1 small head escarole, chopped
Snapper or sea bass, cubed
¼ cup pesto sauce

(*Source: Cooking with California Olive Oil: Treasured Family Recipes* by Gemma Sanita Sciabica)

Halibut with Caper Sauce

❖ ❖ ❖

2 tablespoons drained and roughly chopped capers
¼ cup chopped cornichon pickles
2 hard-cooked eggs, peeled and finely diced
⅓ cup chopped Italian parsley
¼ cup The Olive Press California Mission Extra Virgin Olive Oil

1 tablespoon fresh lemon juice
Salt and pepper to taste
1 cup flour
4 halibut fillets (6–7 ounces each)
2–3 tablespoons vegetable oil
Lemon wedges

Combine the capers, cornichons, eggs, parsley, olive oil, and lemon juice in a bowl. Whisk well so that the egg yolks begin to break down and make the sauce creamier. Season with salt and pepper. Set aside.

Put the flour in a shallow bowl. Season the fish with salt and pepper, then completely dredge it in the flour. Heat 2 tablespoons vegetable oil in a skillet, then add 2 halibut fillets flesh-side down. Cook for about 5 minutes, turn the fish over, and cook another 5 minutes for medium

*Cioppino is a favorite in San Francisco, where it is served with sourdough bread and a bib.

doneness. Transfer to a warmed plate. Repeat with the other 2 fillets, adding more oil to the pan if necessary. Spoon the sauce over the fish and garnish with the lemon wedges. Serves 4.

(*Source:* The Olive Press)

Simple Salmon

❖ ❖ ❖

6 salmon filets (6 ounces each)
1 tomato, peeled, seeded, and
   diced
4 ounces sliced yellow onion
2 ounces sliced carrots
1 lemon, sliced into rounds
2 cloves garlic, sliced
8 ounces vegetable broth

2 ounces olive oil
2 ounces red wine vinegar
2 ounces dry wed wine
2 bay leaves
3 fresh thyme sprigs
4 fresh tarragon leaves
Salt and pepper to taste

Place the 6 salmon filets in an oven-proof glass pan. Add all the other ingredients. Marinate for 1 hour in the refrigerator. In the same glass pan, cover the salmon loosely with a piece of foil and bake for 15 minutes at 350°. When the salmon is done, remove it to a service plate. Strain the liquid from the baking pan and reduce it to less than a cup using a whisk. Adjust the seasonings, and pour the liquid over salmon. Serves 6.

(Recipe created by Chef Salvatore J. Campagna)

Desserts

I remember in the film *Under the Tuscan Sun* when Katherine (Lindsay Duncan) indulges guilt-free in an ice-cream cone and Frances (Diane Lane) takes a peek at the uninhibited woman enjoying herself. It's healthier to eat your favorite foods in moderation than to deprive yourself of life's simple pleasures, which can lead to overeating. While processed cakes, cookies, and ice creams are not healthful (usually because they contain too much sugar, preservatives, and artery-clogging trans fat), homemade desserts can be good for you. Also, any time you can pair fresh fruit with cookies or cake, by all means do as they do in Europe and pile on the best fruit of the season.

Chocolate Chip Oatmeal Cookies
Holiday Carrot Cake
The Olive Press Citrus Cake

Chocolate Chip Oatmeal Cookies

⅓ cup Sciabica Orange Olive Oil
1 large egg
⅓ cup sugar
⅓ cup brown sugar
1 teaspoon vanilla
½ teaspoon Watkins Danish pastry extract
¼ cup orange juice or milk

1 cup flour
¾ cup uncooked quick-cooking oats
1 teaspoon baking soda
¼ teaspoon salt
½ cup chocolate chips
¼ cup currants or raisins

Preheat oven to 375°. Spray a large cookie sheet with non-stick cooking spray. In a mixing bowl, mix the olive oil, egg, sugars, flavorings, and orange juice; stir to blend. Add the flour, oats, baking soda, and salt, and stir until combined. Fold in the chocolate chips and currants.

Drop by level tablespoons (or with a 1-inch ice-cream scooper) 2 inches apart onto Reynolds aluminum (release) foil-lined cookie sheet. Flatten slightly with water-moistened tines of fork.

Bake 12–14 minutes, or until golden brown. Cool on a wire rack. Frost as desired.

(*Source: Cooking with California Olive Oil: Treasured Family Recipes* by Gemma Sanita Sciabica)

Holiday Carrot Cake

❖ ❖ ❖

CAKE

2½ cups all-purpose flour
2 teaspoons baking soda
2 teaspoons cinnamon
¾ teaspoon nutmeg
¾ teaspoon allspice
¾ teaspoon salt

1 cup granulated sugar
¾ cup packed brown sugar
4 eggs
1½ cups extra light olive oil
2½ cups shredded carrots
1 cup walnuts

FROSTING

6 ounces cream cheese, softened
¼ cup butter or margarine, softened
¾ teaspoon vanilla

¼ teaspoon salt
5 cups powdered sugar
2–4 tablespoons half-and-half

Heat oven to 350°. Lightly grease three 9-inch round cake pans with olive oil. Cut waxed paper rounds to fit inside the cake pans.* Grease the waxed paper; lightly flour the pans and liners; set aside.

In a medium bowl, combine the flour, baking soda, cinnamon, nutmeg, allspice, and salt; set aside.

In a mixing bowl, combine the granulated and brown sugars, eggs, and olive oil. Beat at high speed until creamy. Add the carrots and flour mixture. Mix on low speed to moisten. Blend on high speed 1 minute, scraping the sides as needed. Stir in the walnuts. Divide evenly between the prepared pans. Bake 18–22 minutes, or until the top springs back when touched lightly and a wooden pick inserted in the center comes out clean. Cool 10 minutes on cooling racks. Loosen the edges. Remove from the pans; cool completely on the racks.

*To cut waxed paper liners, fold one 30-inch piece of waxed paper into thirds to form a 10-inch piece with 3 layers. Place on the work surface. Place the cake pan on top of the paper and draw around the pan. Use scissors to cut the paper to fit pan, forming 3 liners.

For the frosting: In a mixing bowl, blend the cream cheese, butter, vanilla, and salt. Gradually add the powdered sugar, beating on low speed to mix. Add 2 tablespoons of the half-and-half and beat at high speed, adding the additional half-and-half 1 tablespoon at a time until the desired spreading consistency is reached.

Place 1 cake layer on a serving plate. Reserving about ⅔ of the frosting for the top and sides, spread ½ of the remaining frosting on cake layer. Repeat with another layer. Top with the remaining layer. Frost the top and sides with the reserved frosting. Refrigerate until serving time. Remove the cake from the refrigerator at least 1 hour before serving. Serve at or around room temperature. Serves 12–16.

To make ahead and freeze: Prepare and frost the cake as directed. Freeze 1 hour to firmly set the frosting. Wrap the cake well. Freeze 2–3 days. To serve, remove the cake from the wrapping. Place in a covered cake container in the refrigerator for at least 12 hours. Remove from the refrigerator 2–3 hours before serving.

(*Source:* North American Olive Oil Association)

The Olive Press Citrus Cake

❖ ❖ ❖

Grated zest and juice of 1 lemon
Grated zest and juice of 1 orange
⅓ cup The Olive Press Blood Orange (or The Olive Press Meyer Lemon) Olive Oil
1 cup sugar
¼ teaspoon salt
3 medium eggs

1½ cups semolina
1 cup tightly packed ground almonds
1 teaspoon almond essence
1 teaspoon baking powder
1 teaspoon orange flower water
¼ cup Cointreau or Grand Marnier

Preheat the oven to 325°. Reserve a little of the grated lemon and orange zest, and put the remainder in a bowl with the oil, sugar, salt, orange and lemon juices, and eggs. Beat together with a whisk until light and fluffy and doubled in volume.

Sieve the semolina and baking powder into a second bowl and add the ground almonds. Fold the almond essence and orange flower water into the egg mixture. Pour all at once into the dry ingredients, and fold together, but do not overmix. Spoon into the prepared pan, and smooth the top. Sprinkle the reserved lemon and orange zest over the top.

Bake near the top of the oven for 40–50 minutes, or until pale gold at the edges and firm in the middle. A toothpick inserted into the center should come out clean.

Remove from the oven and let cool in the pan for about 10 minutes. Drizzle the liqueur over the top. Push the cake out, still on the loose metal base, and let it cool on a wire rack for another 10 minutes. Remove the base and paper. Serve in 8–12 wedges, warm or cooled. Do not refrigerate. The cake will keep in an airtight container for up to 4 days.

(*Source:* The Olive Press)

PART 8

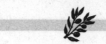

OLIVE OIL RESOURCES

Where Can You Buy Olive Oil?

As olive oil continues to be praised for its powerful health benefits, quality olive oils for the health-conscious and specialty olive oils for olive oil enthusiasts are popping up everywhere around the globe. Currently, a wide world of oils can be bought in supermarkets, specialty stores, and health food stores, as well as through mail order and the Internet. And yes, the decision regarding which one is best can be subjective, just like when choosing your favorite dog breed. Remember, both pure, quality olive oils and canines are judged in the real world.

Here is a list of olive oils, and other types of oils, from organic and natural to commercial brands. If you're interested in buying any of these popular oils and can't find them locally, just contact the manufacturers directly for the locations of stores nearest you.

OLIVE OILS PURCHASED IN RETAIL OUTLETS

Bertolli USA Inc.
300 Hammond Meadow Boulevard
Secaucus, NJ 07094-3621

Olive Oils.

LUCINI PREMIUM SELECT EXTRA VIRGIN OLIVE OIL®
1-888-5LUCINI
www.lucini.com

Lucini Premium Select is a 100 percent Italian extra virgin olive oil produced by Lucini Italia. Olives are a blend of superior Tuscan varieties (primarily the prized Frantoio) grown on private estates in Tuscany's Chianti hills and prime Maremma region. Harvested under the watchful eye of master cultivators—between mid-October and mid-November, when the yield is lower but the quality is highest—olives are pressed within 24 hours in state-of-the-art stainless steel containers.

Lucini's extra virgin, in its distinctive octagonal bottle, is generally available in supermarkets, as well as in selected specialty stores.

Nick Sciabica & Sons
2150 Yosemite Avenue
Modesto, CA 95354
800-551-9612
www.sciabica.com

Sciabica specializes in cold-pressed olive oils using several varieties of California olives. They also provide natural red wine vinegar, as well as balsamic vinegar imported from Modena, Italy.

Since 1936, Sciabica has worked hard to produce the highest quality 100 percent extra virgin olive oil. Sciabica's olive oils have won numerous gold medals from culinary associations, including two gold medals from Chefs in America and one gold medal from the American Tasting Institute, all for "Best of Show."

Sciabica offers a variety of extra virgin olive oils, including:

- *Mission Variety (Winter)*
- *Sevillano Variety (Fall)*
- *Manzanillo Variety (Fall)*
- *Mission Variety Limited*
- *Ascolano Variety (Fall)*
- *Marsala Brand*
- *Kuleto Brand*

Also, Sciabica's "Specialty Olive Oils" include flavored products containing basil, garlic, jalapeño, lemon, and orange. These oils contain no artificial flavors, but are made by crushing and cold-pressing together the ingredients and fresh Mission Variety olives in the mill.

Spectrum Naturals, Inc.
133 Copeland Street
Petaluma, CA 94952
800-995-2705
www.spectrumnaturals.com

Spectrum Naturals (founded in 1986) carries a full line of oils, including unrefined extra virgin olive oil and organic flax oils. (See Part 7 of this book for recipes using Spectrum products.)

Spectrum Naturals offers a vast variety of olive oils and other products, including:

- *Mediterranean Olive Oil, Extra Virgin, Organic*—An all-purpose olive
- *Artisan Oils*—Derived from a nut oil producer in France. The varieties include Toasted Hazelnut Oil, Organic; Toasted Pumpkin Seed Oil, Organic; and Toasted Walnut Oil, Organic.

OLIVE OIL BEAUTY PRODUCTS

Cali
888-883-CALI
www.calicosmetics.com

Products include "extracts of Italian olive oil," such as Moisturizing Olive Oil Soap and Cali Travel Spa.

L'Olivier
Sonoma, CA 95476
www.lolivier-sonoma.com

A wide array of olive oil–based soaps.

OLIVE OIL MILLS AND PRODUCERS IN CALIFORNIA

Apollo Olive Oil
P.O. Box 1054
Oregon House, CA 95962
530-692-2314
www.apollooliveoil.com

Apollo Olive Oil was tagged as one of the top ten olive oil producers in the world in 2006. The judging panel, I Maestri Oleari, is one of the most noteworthy olive oil tasting organizations in the world. Apollo claims its olive oil contains up to 750 milligrams per liter of polyphenols due to its using a unique milling system. Apollo is one of the few California producers that grow their own trees (about 5000 trees, of 37 varieties, from Spain, Italy, France, and Greece) and process oil in their own mills.

B.R. Cohn Olive Oil Co.
15000 Sonoma Highway
Glen Ellen, CA 95442
707-933-9675
www.brcohn.com

Since its founding in 1990, the B.R. Cohn Olive Oil Company has led the renaissance in California olive oil. Its olive oils are certified "extra virgin" by the California Olive Oil Council.
B.R. Cohn Olive Oil Co. offers:

- *Certified Organic California Extra Virgin Olive Oil:* Crafted from organically farmed olives grown, harvested, and pressed in California under the strictest conditions.
- *California Extra Virgin Olive Oil:* A custom blend called "California gold," it's pressed within hours of harvest to ensure freshness.
- *Balsamic and Herb Dipping Oil:* Fruity extra virgin olive oil and balsamic vinegar, highlighted with garlic, herbs, and spices to create a rich dipping oil and complex flavors. Great as a bread dipper or a marinade, tossed with pasta, or used as a hearty vinaigrette for stronger greens.

California Olive Ranch (COR)
2675 Lone Tree Road
Oroville, CA 95965
530-846-8003
www.californiaoliveranch.com

California Olive Ranch is a 700-acre ranch in Oroville, a Northern California agricultural community near the Sierra Nevada foothills. It boasts over 300,000 trees.

COR offers:

- *Arbequina Extra Virgin Olive Oil*
- *Arbosan Extra Virgin Olive Oil*
- *Estate Reserve Blend*

Frantoio Ristorante and Olive Oil Co.
152 Shoreline Highway
Mill Valley, CA 94941
415-289-5777
www.frantoio.com

Frantoio Ristorante and Olive Oil Co. is the only restaurant in the United States with an in-house, state-of-the-art olive oil production facility. At its Web site you can discover how olive oil is made by taking a virtual tour of the restaurant, and can order its premium Certified California and Tuscan Extra Virgin Olive Oils.

McEvoy Ranch
5935 Red Hill Road
Petaluma, CA 94952
707-778-2307
www.mcevoyranch.com

In Marin County, this ranch has 80 acres of Frantoio to Leccino, with approximately 18,000 trees.

The Olive Press
24724 Arnold Drive
Hwy 121
Sonoma, CA 95476
707-965-4839
www.theolivepress.com

The Olive Press was established in 1995 by Ed Stolman (Lunigiana) and Deborah Rogers (Marquesa), both California olive growers and producers who were inspired by the olive-pressing cooperatives of Italy and Southern France. Dedicated to making only the finest award-winning California extra virgin olive oil in its standout facility designed to meet the custom pressing needs of commercial producers, growers with small harvests, and hobbyists wishing to create "estate" olive oil from homegrown olives. Their state-of-the-art Pieralisi press makes it happen.

The Olive Press Tasting Room and Gift Shop and the online store are dedicated to olives and olive oil. Not only do they offer award-winning California extra virgin olive oils for tasting and purchase, but they sell an array of jars of cured olives, olive oil crackers, olive-themed ceramics, and olive oil storage containers.

The Olive Press also is one of the first to offer an olive oil club. Members receive two bottles of the featured olive oils each quarter. Each shipment includes a description of the olive oils to help identify their characteristics, as well as recipe suggestions.

Pasolivo
8530 Vineyard Drive
Paso Robles, CA 93446
805-227-0186
www.pasolivo.com

Pasolivo olive oil is produced at the family's ranch, located in Paso Robles on California's central coast and boasting over 45 acres of olive trees. Pasolivo is the family's signature olive oil, an estate-grown and cold-pressed extra virgin olive oil made of Tuscan olives grown on the ranch. All of their oils are made in their own olive press.

Their products include:

- *Pasolivo Extra Virgin, Estate Tuscan Blend*—Winner, 2 Gold Medals
- *Meyer Lemon Olive Oil*
- *Orange Olive Oil*
- *Lime Olive Oil*

Round Pond
877 Rutherford Crossroad
Rutherford, CA 94573
888-302-2575
www.roundpond.com

Searching for a Mediterranean-type escape—tours and tastings—with a fascinating olive mill tour and adventure of Round Pond artisanal olive oils and wine vinegars? Discover everything you want to know about olive cultivation, harvest, and production before indulging yourself in a guided tasting that includes locally made bread, cheese, and fresh produce.

OLIVE OIL ONLINE FROM SPAIN, ITALY, GREECE, AND FRANCE

In 1996, Judy Ridgway was appointed by the Italian Mastri Oleari (Masters of Olive Oil) to sit as the first non-Italian judge on the judging panel for the prestigious Leone d'Oro Awards for olive oil. She sat on the panel each year until 2001. She provides these top-notch producers in four European regions but made it clear that it is a difficult choice. "There are so many good ones in each of these countries and all very different. Anyway, I will stick a pin in the lists," she says.

Here are several producers worth writing home about to Mediterranean cuisine lovers and anyone interested in extra virgin olive oil.

France
Castelas
www.castelas.com

Greece
Olive Noire
www.olivenoire.com

Italy
Colonna
www.marinacolonna.it
Frantoio Franci
www.frantoiofranci.it

Spain
Marques de Valdueza
www.marquesdevaldueza.com

OLIVE OIL ONLINE FROM OTHER REGIONS AROUND THE GLOBE

China
Olive Connexions Int'l Pte. Ltd.
7 Maxwell Road
#05-07 MND Complex, Annex B
Singapore 069111
www.oliveconnexions.com

OLIVE OIL LAMPS

Lehman's Lamps
One Lehman Lane
289 Kurzen Road
Dalton, OH 44618
www.lehmans.com

Lehman's carries a full line of modern lamps that burn olive oil and other vegetable oils. To order its 160-page catalog of lamps and much more, contact the company.

OLIVE LEAF TEAS

Olivus Olive Leaf Teas for All of Us
www.olivus.com

Olivus is a company dedicated to the benefits of the olive and its leaf, oil, and fruit. Olive leaf is available in capsule, extract, and tea form. Olive leaf tea is an organic, caffeine-free, natural source of antioxidants shown to fight bacteria and viruses, promote circulation, increase energy, and more.

INFORMATION ON OLIVE OIL

California Olive Oil Council (COOC)
P.O. Box 7520
Berkeley, CA 94707
888-718-9830
www.cooc.com

Looking for past or current news, health questions, and events? You will find it all from this organization established in 1992. The mission of the COOC is to promote the fresh, quality extra virgin olive oils made in California. Through its Seal Certification program, it helps everyone from chefs to restaurants find guaranteed extra virgin olive oils for their kitchens. Its membership also welcomes consumers and olive oil producers.

Texas Olive Oil Council (TOOC)
6907 Old Preston Place
Dallas, Texas 75252
214-325-5787
www.texasoliveoilcouncil.org/home.htm

The Texas Olive Oil Council was founded in 1994 as a nonprofit organization that provides consumers and potential growers with information relative to the olive oil industry. It also promotes the quality standards of olive production.

The purpose of the TOOC is to gather and disseminate information regarding the selection, cultivation, and processing of olives, as well as the production, distribution, and marketing of olive oil. The purpose is also to develop and promote standards for the production and labeling of Texas olive oil and to protect and inform the consumer. Its goal is to successfully cultivate olives in Texas.

International Olive Oil Council (IOOC)
Principe de Vergara 154
28002 Madrid, Spain
www.internationaloliveoil.org

The IOOC is a UN-chartered body that regulates olive oil throughout most of the world, but not in the United States.

The Olive Oil Source
www.oliveoilsource.com

A newsletter with a wealth of information about U.S. olive oil companies, international growers, olive oil sales, health, recipes, and much more.

Australian Olive Oil Association (AOOA)
(03) 9696 2143
www.campobellooil.com

The AOOA represents the importers of olive oil into Australia. It is an observer for Australia at the International Olive Oil Council and is responsible for monitoring, on behalf of the IOOC, the purity and chemical quality of olive oil sold in Australia.

OLIVE OIL MUSEUMS

Adatepe Olive Oil Museum
www.adatepe.com

Opened in 2001, Adatepe Olive Oil Museum is the first and only olive oil museum in Turkey. Its goal is to preserve objects belonging to traditional olive extraction, such as ancient presses, various gadgets, amphora, ancient olive oil lamps, and olive oil soap making equipment, and to display them for the new generations. Adatepe Olive Oil Museum shows visitors that the olive tree has a very deep and rich culture.

The museum is also being kept active for olive oil extraction. Every olive season, it uses its traditional olive mill to show visitors how olive oil is made by stone grinders and hydraulic presses. Because of this, it's believed, the Adatepe Olive Oil Museum deserves the "living museum" title.

Museo dell' Olivo
www.museodellolivo.com

Inaugurated in 1992, the Olive Tree Museum receives more than 30,000 visitors annually. The Olive Tree Museum is an Italian private museum, created to portray the olive tree, symbolic of the Mediterranean.

ADDITIONAL INFORMATION

Experience the Olive Harvest
Umbria, Provincia di Perugia, Italy
www.rogaia.com

Villa La Rogaia is an organic farm that cultivates olive trees, produces the finest extra virgin olive oil, and raises medicinal herbs and fragrant plants. Adopt an olive tree at La Rogaia and get olive oil from your own tree. Or come to La Rogaia for a holiday in November and experience the olive harvest, picking your own olive oil.

As of this writing, I find that more manufacturers and retail outlets could be added to this list. However, because of the surge of interest in olive oil and the varied types of oil to choose from, it is impossible to keep up with all the new companies marketing such products. A wide world of olive oil awaits you and your own personal experiences.

Notes

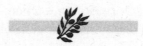

CHAPTER 1:
THE POWER OF OLIVE OIL

1. "Olive Quotes," Food Reference website, www.foodreference.com /html/qolives.html (accessed July 13, 2007).
2. "What Experts Say," The Olive Tree World, www.olivetree.eat-online.net/framehealth.htm (accessed July 13, 2007).
3. Ibid.
4. Liz Applegate, *101 Miracle Foods That Heal Your Heart* (Paramus, NJ: Prentice-Hall Press, 2000), p. 194.

CHAPTER 2:
A GENESIS OF THE OLIVE

1. "Olive Tree Quotes," Food Reference website, www.foodreference. com/html/qolivetrees.html (accessed July 13, 2007).
2. "Rossdhu Olive Oils—Health and Olive Oil," Rossdhu, www.colqu hounolives.com.au/health.html. (accessed July 13, 2007).
3. David Stewart, *Healing Oils of the Bible* (Marble Hill, MO: Care Publications, 2003), p. 97.
4. Ibid., p. 155.
5. "Olive Oil Facts," Pukara Estate, www.pukaraestate.com.au/ Content_Common/pg -Olive-Oil-Facts.seo (accessed July 13, 2007).
6. Ibid.

7. Ibid.
8. Ibid.
9. "The 6,000 Year History of Olive Oil," Filippo Berio, www.filippo berio.com/Tradition/History.asp (accessed July 13, 2007).
10. "Olive Oil Facts," Pukara Estate, www.pukaraestate.com.au/Content Common/pg -Olive-Oil-Facts.seo (accessed July 13, 2007).
11. "The 6,000 Year History of Olive Oil," Filippo Berio, www.filippoberio.com/Tradition/History.asp (accessed July 13, 2007).
12. "Olive Oil," United Nations Conference on Trade and Development, www.unctad.org/infocom/anglais/olive/characteristics.htm (accessed July 13, 2007).
13. "The Olive Tree and Olive Oil in Crete and Greece," Explore Crete, www.explorecrete.com/nature/olive.html (accessed July 13, 2007).

CHAPTER 3:
A HISTORICAL TESTIMONY

1. "The Greek Romance with the Olive," The Hindu Business Line, www.thehindubusinessline.com (accessed July 13, 2007).
2. Charles Quest-Ritson, *Olive Oil* (New York: DK Publishing, 2006), p. 252.
3. http:www.frantoio.com/roberto—christine.htm
4. Frantoio: a dream come true for Roberto and Christina.
5. "Olive Oyl," Wikipedia, http://en.wikipedia.org/wiki/Olive_Oyl (accessed July 13, 2007).

CHAPTER 4:
WHERE ARE THE SECRET INGREDIENTS?

1. "Pleasures of the Table Quotes," Food Reference website, www. foodreference.com/html/qoliveoil.html (accessed July 13, 2007).

CHAPTER 5:
WHY IS OLIVE OIL SO HEALTHY?

1. David Stewart, *Healing Oils of the Bible* (Marble Hill, MO: Care Publications, 2003), p. 159.
2. M. Covas, *Annals of Internal Medicine*, 145 (September 5, 2006), pp. 333–341.
3. David Stewart, *Healing Oils of the Bible*, (Marble Hill, MO: Care Publications, 2003), p. 159.
4. "Effects of Olive Oils in Biomarkers of Oxidative DNA Stress in Northern and Southern Europeans," *The Federation of American Societies for Experimental Biology Journal*, 21 (2007): pp. 45–52.
5. JA Menendez, L Vellon, R Colomer, and R Lupu. "Oleic Acid, the Main Monounsaturated Fatty Acid of Olive Oil, Suppresses Her-2/neu (erbB-2) Expression and Synergistically Enhances the Growth Inhibitory Effects of Trastuzumab (HerceptinTM) in Breast," *Annals of Oncology* (January 10, 2005).
6. David Stewart, *Healing Oils of the Bible*, (Marble Hill, MO: Care Publications, 2003), p. 162.
7. Nikolaos Scarmeas et al., "Mediterranean Diet, Alzheimer Disease, and Vascular Mediation," *Archives of Neurology*, 63 (2006): pp. 1709–77.

CHAPTER 6:
THE KEYS TO THE MEDITERRANEAN DIET

1. "Food Quotes," ThinkExist.com, www.thinkexist.com/quotations/food (accessed July 13, 2007).
2. "The World Health Report 2006," World Health Organization, www.who.int/countries/en (accessed July 13, 2007).
3. *The Journal of the American Medical Association*, February 8, 2006.

CHAPTER 7:
FLAVORED OLIVE OILS

1. "Perfection Quotes," Food Reference website, www.foodreference.com/html/qperfection.html (accessed July 13, 2007).
2. Michael Chiarello, *Flavored Oils and Vinegars: 100 Recipes for*

Cooking with Infused Oils and Vinegars (San Francisco: Chronicle Books, 2006), p. 85.
3. Ibid., p. 85.

CHAPTER 8:
MORE HEALING OILS

1. "What Experts Say," The Olive Tree World, www.olivetree.eat-online.net/framehealth.htm (accessed July 13, 2007).
2. Mary G. Enig, "Flaxseed and Flaxseed Oils for Omega-3 Fatty Acids," The Weston A. Price Foundation for Wise Traditions, www. westonaprice.org/knowyourfats/flaxseed.html (accessed July 13, 2007).

CHAPTER 9:
COMBINING OLIVE OIL AND VINEGAR

1. "Aeschylus," Bartleby.com, www.bartleby.com/66/45/3045.html (accessed July 13, 2007).
2. Jim Long, "Dress for Success," The Herb Companion, www.herb companion.com (accessed July 13, 2007).

CHAPTER 10:
THE ELIXIR TO HEART HEALTH

1. "What Experts Say," The Olive Tree World, www.olivetree.eat-online.net/framehealth.htm (accessed July 13, 2007).
2. Steven Pratt and Kathy Matthews, *SuperFoods Rx: Fourteen Foods That Will Change Your Life* (New York: William Morrow, 2004), p. 112.
3. Editors of FC&A Medical Publishing, *The Folk Remedy Encyclopedia: Olive Oil, Vinegar, Honey and 1,001 Other Home Remedies* (Peachtree City, GA: FC&A Medical Publishing, 2001), p. 168.
4. Ibid.
5. K. Covas, HE. Nyyssonen et al., "The Effect of Polyphenols in Olive Oil on Heart Disease Risk Factors." *Annals of Internal Medicine 145* (2006): pp. 333–341.
6. Katherine Esposito et al., "Effect of a Mediterranean-Style Diet

on Endothelial Dysfunction and Markers of Vascular Inflammation in the Metabolica Syndrome," *Journal of the American Medical Association*, 292 (September 22–29, 2004): pp. 1440-1446.

CHAPTER 11:
THE OLIVE OIL DIET

1. "What Experts Say," The Olive Tree World, www.olivetree.eat-online.net/framehealth.htm (accessed July 13, 2007).
2. Seth Roberts, *The Shangri-La Diet: The No Hunger Eat Anything Weight-Loss Plan* (New York: Putnam, 2006), p. 30.
3. Ibid., p. 31.

CHAPTER 12:
ANTIAGING WONDER FOOD

1. "Olive Oil Quotes," Food Reference website, www.foodreference.com/html/qoliveoil.html (accessed July 13, 2007).

CHAPTER 13:
CURES FROM YOUR KITCHEN

1. "The Olive Tree and Olive Oil in Crete and Greece," Explore Crete, www.explorecrete.com/nature/olive.html (accessed July 13, 2007).

CHAPTER 14:
OLIVE OIL MANIA: USING OLIVE OIL FOR THE HOUSEHOLD, KIDS, PETS, AND BEAUTY

1. "Hemingway, Ernest," Bartleby.com, www.bartleby.com (accessed July 13, 2007).
2. Carol Firenze, *The Passionate Olive: 101 Things to Do with Olive Oil* (New York: Ballantine Books, 2005), p. 144.
3. Ibid., p. 148.
4. Ibid., p. 145.

CHAPTER 15:
OLIVE BEAUTIFUL

1. "Olive Branch Quotes," ThinkExist.com, www.thinkexist.com/quotations/food (accessed July 13, 2007).

CHAPTER 16:
OLIVE OIL PRODUCERS, TASTING BARS, AND TOURS

1. "Olive Oil Quotes," Food Reference website, www.foodreferences.com/html/qoliveoil.html (accessed July 13, 2007).
2. Charles Quest-Ritson, *Olive Oil* (New York: DK Publishing, 2006), p. 135.
3. Ibid, p. 53.
4. Ibid, p. 227.

CHAPTER 17:
OLIVE OIL IS NOT FOR EVERYONE: SOME BITTER VIEWS

1. "Olive Oil Quotes," ThinkExist.com, www.thinkexist.com (accessed July 13, 2007).

CHAPTER 18:
THE JOY OF COOKING WITH OLIVE OIL

1. RoeValenti and Cal Orey, *Just Cook It! How to Get Culinary Fit . . . 1-2-3* (Lincoln, NE: iUniverse, 2004), p. 50.
2. Ibid.
3. Michel Stroot, *The Golden Door Spa Cooks Light & Easy* (Layton, UT: Gibbs Smith, 2003).

Selected Bibliography

Baird, Pat. *The Pyramid Cookbook: Pleasures of the Food Guide Pyramid.* New York: Henry Holt and Company, 1994.

Bickers, Merry. *I Didn't Know That Olive Oil Would Burn!* Self-published, 1997.

Cooper, Ann. *Lunch Lessons: Changing the Way We Feed Our Children.* New York: HarperCollins, 2006.

Firenze, Carol. *The Passionate Olive.* New York: Ballantine Books, 2005.

Haas, Elson. *Staying Healthy with Nutrition, 21st Century Edition.* Berkeley, CA: Celestial Arts, 2006.

Keys, Ancel and Margaret Keys. *How to Eat Well and Stay Well the Mediterranean Way.* New York: Doubleday, 1975.

Krasner, Deborah. *The Flavors of Olive Oil: A Tasting Guide and Cookbook.* New York: Simon & Schuster, 2002.

Orey, Cal. *Magic of Oils, Scents and Candles.* Boca Raton, FL: American Media, 2000.

Orey, Cal. *Doctors' Orders: What 101 Doctors Do to Stay Healthy.* New York: Kensington, 2002.

Orey, Cal. *The Healing Powers of Vinegar: A Complete Guide to Nature's Most Remarkable Remedy,* revised and updated. New York: Kensington, 2006.

Orey, Cal and Mark Jabo. *The Sky is Falling! A Global Warming Survival Guide.* Bloomington, IN: AuthorHouse, 2006.

Ridgway, Judy. *Judy Ridgway's Best Olive Oil Buys 'Round the World.* New York: Gardiner Press, 2005.

Roberts, Seth. *The Shangri-La Diet: The No Hunger Eat Anything Weight-Loss Plan*. New York: Putnam, 2006.

Sciabica, Gemma Sanita. *Baking with California Olive Oil: Dolci and Biscotti Recipes*. Modesto, CA: Gemma Sanita Sciabica, 1997.

Sciabica, Gemma Sanita. *Cooking with California Olive Oil: Treasured Family Recipes*. Modesto, CA: Gemma Sanita Sciabica, 1998.

Sciabica, Gemma Sanita. *Cooking with California Olive Oil: Popular Recipes*. Modesto, CA: Gemma Sanita Sciabica, 2001.

Sciabica, Gemma Sanita. *Baking Sensational Sweets with California Olive Oil*. Modesto, CA: Gemma Sanita Sciabica, 2005.

Sears, Barry. *Enter the Zone: A Dietary Road Map*. New York: Regan Books, 1995.

Simopoulos, Artemis P., *The Omega Diet: The Lifesaving Nutritional Program Based on the Diet of the Island of Crete*. New York: HarperCollins, 1998.

Wolke, Robert L. *What Einstein Told His Cook: Kitchen Science Explained*. New York: W.W. Norton & Company, 2005.